Living with Parkinson's

Also by David Carroll
with the Brookdale Center on Aging

When Your Loved One Has Alzheimer's

Living with Parkinson's

A GUIDE FOR THE PATIENT AND CAREGIVER

DAVID L. CARROLL

Based on methods developed by the
Brookdale Center on Aging

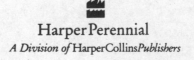

HarperPerennial
A Division of HarperCollins*Publishers*

A hardcover edition of this book was published in 1992 by HarperCollins Publishers.

First HarperPerennial edition published 1993.

Designed by Alma Orenstein

The Library of Congress has catalogued the hardcover edition as follows:
Carroll, David, 1942–
    Living with Parkinson's : a guide for the patient and caregiver /
David L. Carroll.—1st ed.
        p.   cm.
    "Based on methods developed by the Brookdale Center on Aging."
    Includes bibliographical references and index.
    ISBN 0-06-016159-0 (cloth)
    1. Parkinsonism—Popular works. I. Brookdale Center on Aging (Hunter College).
    II. Title. [DNLM: 1. Activities of Daily Living—popular works. 2. Antiparkinson Agents—popular works. 3. Exercise Therapy—popular works. 4. Parkinson Disease—drug therapy—popular works. 5. Parkinson Disease—rehabilitation—popular works. WL   359   C319L]
RC382.C39   1992
616.8'33—dc20
DNLM/DLC
for Library of Congress   91-50475

ISBN 0-06-092367-9 (pbk.)
93 94 95 96 97 CW 10 9 8 7 6 5 4 3 2 1

Contents

PART II
Physical Activity and PD: A Practical Guide

PART III
Everyday Hints for Living with Parkinson's Disease

Acknowledgments

Thanks and gratitude to the following persons for their help with this book: Dr. William Barrett, Dr. Jon Dorman, Dr. Della Williams, Dr. Ray Vickers, Dr. Seyed Abdulla, Dr. Hermin Liprit, Dr. Ralph Sachs; also to Barbara Lee, Barbara Barry, Jane Goldberg, Ellen Greenfield, Lisa Rindoni, Phil Toombs, Rice Lorimor, Phyllis Jacobson; June Carroll, Ali Rodell, Brynn Carroll, Layla Carroll, Hannah Harrison, John Matarazzo; Dr. Rose Dobrof, Dr. Harry Moody, Marilyn Howard, and many others at the Brookdale Center; Rena Orner, Libby Fine, Bill Auld, Jim and Nancy Barberio, Betty and Jim Bennett, Pat and Peggy Burke, Jerry and Martha Donovan, Jeanette and Leonard Elkin, Dave and Helen Fisher, Irving and Rhoda Greenberg, Marie Kantrowitz, Joe and Helen Knizek, Les and Anita Lilien, Olga Livsey, Allan and Dorothy Magrino, Fred and Esther Martin, John and Betty McCormach, Marie and Arthur Reilly, Robert and Genevieve Reim, Marilyn and Bob Sormani, and with extra special thanks to Mary Jane Derven, Juan and Jean Nickford, Ed and Priscilla Haines, Betty and Jim Monaghan, Lucille Ferretti, and Max Feller—may they all prosper.

Introduction

SO YOU HAVE PARKINSON'S DISEASE

So you have Parkinson's disease. Well, you are in good company. Approximately 1 million other Americans wake up every morning knowing they have the same disorder. Perhaps your condition has recently been diagnosed and you wish to find out more about it. Perhaps you are experiencing Parkinson's-like symptoms and are seeking more information on the subject. Perhaps you have had this ailment for some time and wish to learn what you can do to live with your handicaps and to maximize your assets. Or maybe you are the caregiver and/or a relative of a person who suffers from this difficult disease and are anxious to be of service.

Whatever the case, there will most likely be something in these pages to help you. Because Parkinson's disease, or "PD" as many people call it, is a disease that *can* be helped. It is one of the few chronic neurological ailments for which there now exists: (1) effective medications, (2) rehabilitative physical therapy, and (3) efficient practical aids for daily living. All of these therapeutic supports really work, and all really do help patients achieve a quality of life that in many cases approaches the normal.

The first of these benefits, medication, is clearly the most important of the three and is the one that you probably know the most about from speaking with your doctor. In the pages that follow we will discuss this subject in detail.

Physical therapy is not as frequently spoken about in the doctor's office, and as a rule patients must seek out a physical therapist or a PD support group to learn more about the exercises that help the stiffness associated with PD.

The third item, the practical aids for the activities of daily living, are rarely discussed at all in the doctor's office or in any formal medical facility for that matter. Doctors are busy men and women who usually have time only to prep you in the things they know best, namely, diagnosis and chemical medication. The rest is left up to you.

And yet, the fact remains that to derive the maximum benefit from a therapeutic plan for PD, a three-way balance must be achieved between medication, physical activity, and aids for daily living. Therefore:

1. In Part I of this book we will discuss PD medications in detail: how they work, what they cost, dosages, schedules, tricks, what they do and don't do, and what to expect from their use.

2. In Part II the subject of physical therapy will be profiled, with emphasis on exercise programs, building stamina and energy, therapeutic equipment, vitamins, diet, and speech therapy.

3. Finally, in Part III we will discuss the activities of daily living. This section will provide experience-proven advice concerning the daily problems that PD persons face: getting in and out of a chair or the front seat of a car; holding a mixing bowl with a shaking hand; writing when one's writing hand cramps; getting "unstuck" when one freezes; finding the right pair of shoes to support weakened ankles; brushing one's hair when it's hard to get a grip on the brush; and many, many more nitty-gritty concerns of ordinary living that are faced by persons with PD every hour of the day.

The information in the pages that follow, it should be added, the medical advice, the case histories, interviews, quotes, and references come mostly from work with professionals and patients affiliated with New York City's Brookdale Center on Aging. Let's get acquainted.

MEET THE BROOKDALE CENTER ON AGING

The Brookdale Center on Aging, located adjacent to Bellevue Hospital in downtown Manhattan, is affiliated with Hunter College and with the City University of New York. One of the largest and best known geriatric facilities in the world, the Brookdale Center concerns itself with a remarkably wide spectrum of issues in the field of aging including the legal rights of senior citizens, ethical dilemmas in medicine, caregiving for the aged, intergenerational programs for young and old, and geriatric education.

Over the years one of the most pressing priorities for Brookdale has been to sponsor methods of care for older persons who suffer from chronic, debilitating diseases. Long a leader in the field of Alzheimer's disease and related dementia, Brookdale concerns itself with other major disorders of the elderly as well, Parkinson's disease among them, and many of the professionals associated with, or friendly to, Brookdale are expert in this field.

Working hand-in-hand with Brookdale's staff and with medical professionals and self-help groups, the author conducted a number of on-site interviews with neurologists, nurses, physical therapists, occupational therapists, speech therapists, and perhaps most importantly, patients who suffer from Parkinson's disease. A majority of the facts, opinions, and advice presented in these pages is taken from these conversations, as well as from the latest medical information provided by Brookdale's staff of library affiliates.

This book, in essence, owes its existence to Brookdale and to the generosity of its staff. My thanks to this benevolent organization for their support, council, and cooperation, and for the many efforts they have made through the years to aid and improve health care for the growing population of elderly people in our country.

PART I

All About Parkinson's Disease

1

What Is Parkinson's Disease?

WHAT IS PARKINSON'S DISEASE?

Parkinson's disease is a syndrome of symptoms, the most prevalent being tremor of the limbs or head, postural instability, muscular rigidity, a decrease in spontaneous movements, and a general slowing of a patient's overall physical and emotional affect. It was discovered—*recognized* is a better term, perhaps—by the English physician and writer of political diatribes, James Parkinson, who in 1817 penned a seminal tract on the subject entitled *Essay on the Shaking Palsy*. In this paper he presented a fairly complete description of what up till that time had been known simply as "the shaking."

> Involuntary tremulous motion, with lessened muscular power, in parts not in action and even when supported; with a propensity to bend the trunk forward, and to pass from a walking to a running pace; the senses and intellect being uninjured.

This compact list of observations called attention to the interconnectedness of such symptoms as gait disorder, tremor, and postural leaning, and for the first time in history suggested that they constituted a single chronic disease. Dr. Parkinson's description is, in fact, touted as a masterpiece of neurologic definition, and experts in the field will assure you that few medical observers have improved on its concision.

What causes Parkinson's disease? No one knows for sure. All that is understood about its etiology at this time is that certain sets of cells in the brain begin to degenerate, and that this decay produces the syndrome of symptoms we call parkinsonism.

The forces that trigger this apparently unprovoked carnage of brain cells are mysterious and as yet untraceable. Some experts believe that the degenerative process is started—or at least accelerated—by toxic substances in the environment. We know, for instance, that laborers who work with manganese occasionally come down with Parkinson's-like symptoms; and that people who live in cities have PD more frequently than do occupants of rural areas (it has likewise been noted that persons in rural areas who develop parkinsonism tend to live in places where chemical pesticides and fertilizers are common).

Other medical researchers maintain that an unknown and unidentified virus is at the heart of the disorder. As evidence, they point to the great flu epidemic of 1916 that caused many of its victims to develop symptoms that are undeniably Parkinson's-like in their appearance.

Still other experts in the field claim that PD is simply the result of accelerated aging, that certain cells in the brain die off as a matter of course, and that any man or woman who happens to live to a ripe enough old age will develop this ailment as a matter of course. There are many theories, but no certainties.

Is the disease inherited? Medical opinions are divided on this matter too, though most genetic studies indicate that persons with a family history of PD are *slightly* more apt to develop it than those without such a history—but only slightly, and even this finding is in dispute. All in all, if a member of your family suffers from PD you probably shouldn't spend a good deal of time worrying about it. If the disorder has any genetic component at all the risk factor is likely to be so small that, statistically speaking, the odds are overwhelmingly in your favor that you will not inherit the disease.

There are several other interesting and puzzling elements about Parkinson's. For example, more white people develop it than black. More westerners get it than orientals, and slightly more men than women show symptoms before the age of sixty (though after sixty the curve flattens out, with the frequency rate becoming equal for both sexes). While the disease predominantly strikes people who have passed their sixtieth year, many individuals have gotten it in their forties and fifties, and the numbers of young victims developing the disorder is on the dramatic rise. Why this increase no one knows, though it seems likely that our industrialized, toxified environment contributes in some way to this alarming phenomenon.

DOPAMINE

All in all, much of what we know concerning the origins and antecedents of Parkinson's disease is conjectural. But if its essential cause is a stubbornly kept secret of nature, we do possess a good deal of knowledge concerning the process that occurs in the body once it begins. Reducing this process to a simplified model, it works something like this.

Among the many chemical substances that activate the brain, the so-called *neurotransmitters* are among the most crucial. Neurotransmitters are chemical messenger substances produced by nerve cells. Once manufactured, these substances stimulate the sending of microelectric signals/information from neuron to neuron, keeping the entire network of nerve cell units interconnected, and helping the unfathomably complex arabesque of nerves and ganglia we call the nervous system to function as a single grand unity.

One of the most important neurotransmitters produced by the human organism is called *dopamine*. This critical substance plays several key roles in the body including that of hormonal trigger (it helps activate adrenaline and noradrenaline, thus overseeing the human "fight or flight" mechanism), a regulator of daily mood, and a controlling factor in motor movement and coordination.

The cells that produce dopamine are located deep in the brain, in the basal ganglia area in general and in the sector of the brain known as the *substantia nigra* in particular. Dark and pigmented (hence its name meaning "black substance" in Latin), the substantia nigra is in turn connected to other parts of the basal ganglia by a network of long nerve fibers that twist and turn gracefully beneath the hemispheres of the brain like an underground plant with spidery roots. After the dopamine is manufactured in the substantia nigra it is sent along these fibers to its final destination, the *corpus striatum,* where it will perform its duties as a transmitter of neurological impulses, helping in the regulation of muscular response and overall body function.

Now at any given time day or night dopamine cells in the substantia nigra are being destroyed. At this very moment, perhaps, several are disintegrating in your own brain due, let us say, to a prior head injury, or to toxins, air pollutants, the natural process of aging, or whatever. But don't be alarmed. In its typical profusion nature has created so many of these cells that enormous numbers can perish before harmful effects occur. It is estimated, in fact, that over three-quarters of our dopamine-producing cells can be eliminated before the body begins to show a visible response.

And yet with Parkinson's disease, for reasons unknown, this is exactly what occurs. So many of the dopamine-making cells in the substantia nigra become damaged that gradually, inevitably, smaller and smaller amounts of dopamine reach the corpus striatum, until eventually parkinsonian symptoms begin to appear. Even the excesses of biologic creation have not produced enough of these cells to withstand the destruction. Parkinson's disease has begun.

PROGNOSIS

What will happen to people with PD? How sick will they become? Is the disease fatal?

In a word, no. It is not a fatal disease; not anymore. With the advent of L-dopa and other important PD medications, the progress of PD can now be forestalled for so long that a majority of patients live out their normal life span.

Will PD produce handicaps? Yes. But just *how* handicapped a person will become is impossible to say. For though PD is known to be a degenerative disease, the speed at which it develops is different for each individual. Some patients, for example, become severely handicapped after a decade or less. Others continue for fifteen, twenty, even twenty-five years with relatively few increases in their symptoms. There are no certainties in this department.

The development of parkinsonism, moreover, is not always predictably progressive; that is, simply because a symptom is bad today does not mean it will be bad tomorrow. It may improve tomorrow, and the day after that too. Or vice versa. It is difficult to say. PD, in other words, does not necessarily move from good to bad to worse to worst. It sometimes hopscotches, as it were, going from bad, to good, to better, to worse, to so-so, and back again to good. PD is not necessarily a linear disease, as is made clear by these Parkinsonian patients:

Lee G.: You never know. I thought my tremor had progressed to the point of my being unable to use my hand. Then it got a lot better; why I don't know. Parkinson's disease is like a roller coaster—you never know when you're going to go up or when you're going to go down.

Thelma A.: My condition has stabilized over the past years. I wouldn't say I've gotten any worse over the past seven years since I got the disease. In the first years I felt like I was falling down a well—things were getting bad so fast. It was out of control. Then all of a sudden it seemed my symptoms stabilized and have stayed at the same plateau since, no better and no worse.

Thatcher B.: The first thing I asked my doctor when I found out I had Parkinson's disease was "How long do I got, Doc?" He looked at me and laughed. "As long as the rest of us," he said. "You'll just have to keep your safety belt a little more tightly buckled for the ride."

Margaret O.: You take it a day at a time. An hour at a time. You thank God you're doing as well as you are. You try not to think about what will happen tomorrow, cause no one can know that. If you think about that kind of thing too much your imagination gets the better of you. I have Parkinson's disease now, that's all I know, and when I look around at other persons my age with all kinds of terrible diseases, like Alzheimer's disease and cancer, I am thankful that I'm doing as well as I am. I am really thankful. Parkinson's disease is not so bad as far as serious diseases go.

PERSPECTIVES

In the long run, there are two ways of looking at PD, both of which must be understood if one is to gain a complete view of the disease. The first is shared by individuals who do not actually suffer from the disease but who know a great deal about its cause, care, and treatment. Into this category fall physicians, various medical professionals, and caregivers. All have a good deal to offer you, the reader, by way of information, observation, and advice.

The second perspective belongs to the patients themselves. These brave men and women often know a good deal about the physiology and biochemistry of their disease. They tend to be a remarkably well-informed lot. But whether or not they can tell you what dopamine is, or what the corpus striatum does in the neural network, they have a kind of knowledge that nonpatients do not: the knowledge gained from experience.

They know, for example, what it means to flounder about for twenty minutes in the middle of the night struggling to turn over in bed. Or how it feels to find themselves stuck in a chair and to be unable to stand up in the middle of a formal social occasion. They know the embarrassment of drooling in front of strangers.

They know what it means to force their bodies to move when their bodies insist on staying inert; to speak when their voice has less force in it than a sigh; to undergo heroic acts of will simply to accomplish tasks that healthy people take for granted. They know what it means to wrestle with adversity and to survive.

With the help of the Brookdale Center and of several other facilities in the New York metropolitan area, many of these patients and their caregivers will now be heard from loudly and clearly in the pages that follow. These determined men and women have a great deal to tell all of us, not only about Parkinson's disease itself, but about living with struggle and overcoming the odds. It is to these special people—and particularly to the men and women of the Nyack Hospital Parkinson's support group—that this book is humbly dedicated. Dauntless individuals all, they are in my opinion and in the opinion of many other sage observers, the proponents, par excellence, of what the great Dr. Johnson was speaking of when he remarked that "To seize the good that is within our reach—that is the great art of life." It is the great art of living with PD as well.

GLOSSARY OF PARKINSON'S TERMS

Acetylcholine: An important *neurotransmitter* adversely affected in Parkinson's disease patients.

Agonist: A chemical that enhances the action of a *neurotransmitter*.

Akinesia: Slowness of body movement, similar to *bradykinesia*.

Amantadine: A common Parkinson's medication known commercially as Symmetrel.

Anticholinergic drug: A type of Parkinson's medication that opposes the body's production of *acetylcholine* and keeps the acetylcholine in balance with the body's *dopamine* supplies.

Basal ganglia: A large gray area in the lower central part of the brain that helps control motor movements and that is afflicted in persons with PD.

Bradykinesia: Slowness of physical movement.

Bromocriptine: A newly developed Parkinson's medication that acts as an *agonist* to fool the dopamine receptors.

Carbidopa: A substance that inhibits the breakdown of *L-dopa* in the system and is an essential ingredient in the drug *Sinemet.*

Cogwheeling rigidity: A type of muscular *rigidity* that produces a ratcheted, cogwheel-like resistance in the limbs of Parkinson's patients.

Corpus striatum: A section of the *basal ganglia* that receives *dopamine* supplies from the *substantia nigra.*

Dementia: A condition of lowered or retarded mental acuteness.

Deprenyl: A newly developed medication for Parkinson's disease that acts by inhibiting an enzyme that destroys *dopamine.*

Dopamine: A basic *neurotransmitter,* a deficit of which is responsible for producing the symptoms of *parkinsonism.*

Dyskinesia: Uncontrolled writhing movements of the limbs and/or body produced as a side effect of certain Parkinson's medications.

Festinating gait: A shuffling type of walk characteristic of persons with Parkinson's.

Ideopathic Parkinson's: The most common type of *parkinsonism.* Ideopathic means "of unknown origin."

L-dopa: An amino acid that is used in Parkinson's medication to restore supplies of *dopamine* to the brain and hence restore normal functioning.

Levodopa: A form of *L-dopa.*

Livedo reticularis: A mottled condition of the skin that results from long-term use of the drug *amantadine.*

Micrographia: Handwriting that becomes smaller as it runs across the page, a typical symptom of Parkinson's patients.

MPTP: A toxic chemical that produces Parkinson's-like symptoms in its users.

Neuroleptic drug: A tranquilizer type of drug such as Thorazine that occasionally produces symptoms of *parkinsonism.*

Neurotransmitter: A chemical substance in the brain that is responsible for the transmission of chemical/electrical messages from neuron to neuron.

On-off syndrome: A tendency among Parkinson's patients to become suddenly fatigued and immobile due to the fading affects of medication.

Parkinsonism: A clinical condition characterized by *tremor, rigidity,* and *bradykinesia.*

Rigidity: A basic symptom of *parkinsonism* characterized by stiffness in the muscles and limbs.

Sinemet: A Parkinson's drug composed of L-dopa mixed with *carbidopa.* It is generally considered to be the most effective PD medication.

Substantia nigra: A section of the *basal ganglia* responsible for producing *dopamine.*

Tremor: A basic symptom of *parkinsonism* characterized by a slow, four- to seven-second rhythmical shaking of the limbs, head, or other parts of the body.

2

Is It Parkinson's?

Lisa Roberts has been out of sorts for some time. No particular diagnosis, no debilitating symptoms. Just, as she describes it, "a feeling of not being myself."

Every day Lisa drives to work at a local elementary school, makes supper for her husband Jerry, visits friends, and plays backgammon with her sister—a regular round of social and family affairs. Everything seems normal. And yet something is wrong, of this Lisa is intuitively sure.

It has to do with her energy level most of all. A robust woman in her late fifties, Lisa normally plays tennis twice a week after work and hikes with members of a conservation and ecology club on Saturdays. Over the past several months, however, she has started missing her tennis appointments and has been absent five weekends in a row from the club outings. Friends called to ask if anything is wrong.

"I'm not really sure," Lisa replied. "I thought I had the flu for a while. Or arthritis. Whatever it is, it doesn't want to go away."

Several people asked about her exact symptoms.

"I feel uncomfortable all the time," Lisa answered. "My muscles ache, in my back and hip especially. I'm tired a lot, especially after I walk, and I don't feel so steady on my feet. I've even lost my balance a couple of times. It takes twice as long to get things done."

"Do you feel down, depressed?" a close associate at school asked her.

"I wouldn't call it depressed," Lisa answered. "It's more like being—uneasy. Ill at ease. Just—how can I say it—as if something inside me is tightening up. I'm simply not my normal self."

Lisa's friends and family urged her to see a doctor. But she was reluctant. "It will pass," she told her well wishers. "It's just one of those viruses."

But it didn't pass, and gradually Lisa's condition became increasingly obvious. People noticed that her posture was becoming subtly stooped, something uncharacteristic of Lisa who exercised regularly. She seemed to take less interest in things around her. Most alarming was the fact that her face was taking on a kind of bland, masklike expression during much of the day, even in moments of excitement. "It's like something out of the movie *The Invasion of the Body Snatchers*, Lisa's husband confided to his doctor. Lisa's body is here, her voice is here, her face—but is Lisa inside anymore? I don't know."

Finally, after family and friends pleaded with her to seek help, Lisa made an appointment with her doctor. Several weeks after her first visit she was diagnosed as having Parkinson's disease.

THE INSIDIOUS ONSET

Lisa's story is less common than others, perhaps, because her condition was not typified by major Parkinson's symptoms. In Frank R.'s case, a slight but persistent manual tremor interfered with his work as a dentist and sent him to seek professional help. Rita G. experienced an uncharacteristic stiffness when she worked in her garden, and after months of discomfort decided it was cause for concern.

Lisa's story is quite typical in other ways, however. First, she was reluctant to take her symptoms seriously, a trait that many early PD people display; second, her visit to the doctor was delayed and ultimately not self-initiating; third, like practically every PD sufferer, her condition came on in imperceptible degrees. It "sneaked up on me like a thief in the night," she told a friend.

Insidious is the medical term used to describe this type of symptomatic onset. Derived from the Latin verb meaning "to ambush," the word implies something stealthy and silent, a disease (as *Taber's Cyclopedic Medical Dictionary* defines it) "that comes on imperceptibly and does not necessarily exhibit early symptoms of its advent."

For this reason persons may experience a number of seemingly small physical debilities without realizing that any of them are connected to PD. In the first popular book written on PD, *Parkinson's Disease,* Dr. Roger Duvoisin remarks that he spotted early signs of Parkinson's disease in a patient by watching the patient's movements in an old home movie. This event, Duvoisin remarks, occurred five or six years before the person was actually diagnosed. In another instance, Duvoisin says, many years before the obvious onset of PD, a woman patient was consulting a speech therapist about her "mumbly voice."[1]

THE RELUCTANT DIAGNOSIS

The indiscernible arrival and unhurried development of Parkinson's disease is what allows patients to live with the disorder for months and even years before receiving a formal medical diagnosis. People may experience a certain slowness of movement, a slight shaking of the hand, increased stiffness, a drop in energy level, and chalk it all off to the passing years. What's more, they may be right. Many of the early signs of PD are similar to those brought on by normal aging.

Thus, doctors may be unwilling to categorically diagnose Parkinson's disease until a recognizable symptomatic picture emerges. A man or woman suffering from minor complaints such as backache or stiff neck may be treated by specialists for years before anyone realizes the true cause of the problem. Dr. Robert Barrett, a neurologist in private practice in New York City, says:

> I remember one time there was a doctor who I treated down in central Delaware. This man went first to an orthopedic surgeon because his wrist was persistently sore. He thought he had tendonitis. The doctor there started giving him injections. These worked sometimes and sometimes they didn't, but over time his wrist just kept getting stiffer and stiffer. Meanwhile, there was no indication of other symptoms involved, no tremor or anything else during all this time, and the condition continued this way for years until other symptoms did start to appear and we realized that Parkinson's disease was the true underlying pathology behind this man's problems.

Because the disease is controllable but not curable, an early diagnosis of PD is not necessarily of vital importance. If the complaints are not developed enough to seriously bother the patient, they may not warrant chemical palliation either. There is, in fact, some evidence (that is hotly debated among professionals, it should be added) to indicate that when PD medications are prescribed too soon they *speed up* the progress of the disease rather than retard it.

Because of the undefined character of early symptoms, moreover, many people avoid seeking medical consultation of any kind. Aside from the common knowledge that tremor and Parkinson's disease are somehow associated, and despite the fact that several world-class celebrities such as Muhammad Ali and Katharine Hepburn exhibit forms of Parkinson's, the disease's telltale signals are not widely recognized and its symptoms do not have the dramatic public familiarity as do those of, say, Alzheimer's disease. People suffering from undiagnosed PD may therefore sense that something is wrong or out of whack, but since they know little about parkinsonism and are not yet uncomfortable enough to seek professional help, they maintain the status quo.

Quite understandable. Denial is a form of self-protection we all invoke at one time or another. The problem is that untreated complaints can eventually interfere with normal functioning. A tremor may cause an office assistant to make unnecessary typing errors. Increased stiffness prevents a bricklayer from climbing up and down a ladder. Such troubles, moreover, become psychologically harassing as well as physically irritating, and eventually sufferers get caught in a hellish limbo between worry and denial, inventing convenient and often wildly inaccurate medical scenarios to explain their problems. Ignorance is clearly not bliss in such cases, and at a certain point a visit to the physician becomes the wisest choice, even if a person's symptoms *seem* to be minor. What exactly are these symptoms?

WHEN TO SUSPECT PARKINSON'S

There are three major physical symptoms that characterize PD:

1. Tremor
2. Muscular rigidity
3. Increased slowness of motion, a condition known medically as *akinesia* or more commonly, *bradykinesia*

Generally, though not inevitably, people must exhibit at least two of these three symptoms for a diagnosis of Parkinson's disease to be made. There are a number of lesser complaints that may accompany them as well and these will be discussed below.

Note that not all three symptoms may occur in the early days of PD. One PD sufferer, a beauty technician who works at a hair salon in Chicago, experienced slight trembling of her right hand approximately twice a week, usually when she was in the midst of preparing a difficult coiffure. The shaking caused her so little trouble and tended to arrive at such widely spaced intervals that for a while she thought of it simply as "nerves."

Sometimes an early symptom such as a tremor will occur by itself and will not be joined by a second major symptom, muscular rigidity, say, or a third, like bradykinesia, for years to come. In certain cases, symptoms two and three never come at all.

Usually, however, they do come, and diagnosing PD at this

point is often definitive. Those who suspect Parkinson's should thus be on the alert for these initial symptoms and should observe them carefully if they come, gathering as much data as possible for future reporting to a physician. Here is how these three characteristic symptoms present themselves.

Tremor

Because it is at once highly visible and annoyingly incapacitating, tremor is the complaint that most frequently causes people to seek medical counsel. The most common of Parkinson's symptoms, it afflicts approximately 75 percent of the PD population and is often the first indication of the disease. Not atypically, a person will notice a faint shake in one hand or foot—rarely in both. The shaking may be felt in the neck, mouth, or jaw (not in the whole head, as is commonly believed) or in the stomach or chest. Produced by alternating contractions of antagonistic muscle groups, the tremor is involuntary and intermittent, especially in the beginning, and obeys no apparent timetable. Fortunately, the early tremor of most PD patients disappears during sleep.

In the beginning most people find that their shaking is confined to one side of the body, though more than one limb may be involved. When Jim B. first showed signs of PD his left hand shook for a few minutes, stopped, then his left foot took over. In time, a kind of rhythmic alternation developed between hand and foot.

When an early tremor is exclusively localized in the hand, as it often is, it produces a "pill-rolling" motion that makes it appear that the person is shaping a pill or small piece of clay between the thumb and fingers (upon close examination the finger movements are actually more parallel than rotary). Tremors often appear first in one or two fingers, a thumb, or a single toe.

Characteristically, a PD tremor remains quiescent when the limb is in motion (as when reaching for a cup), then starts up again when the limb slows down or comes to a rest (as when the cup is brought to the lips in the static drinking position). Many PD people notice that purposeful activity such as lifting, carrying, pushing, or using an arm to swing a tennis racket or a hammer causes the tremor to stop, and that it begins again as soon as the limb ceases its exertions. Because of this peculiarity some PD patients intentionally put their hands in constant motion during conversation, simply to keep the tremor under control. In approximately 15 percent of cases a so-called *action tremor* is present whereby the shaking continues both during activity and rest.

A definite relationship exists between emotions and symptoms, especially concerning the tremor. As any PD patient will tell you, during periods of anxiousness, self-consciousness, or excitement, shaking tends to increase, sometimes dramatically. This is especially true in a crowd or in a demanding social situation. While the severity of emotion-induced shaking can sometimes be lessened by making a conscious effort to relax, such attempts are not always feasible. It is usually not until the person returns to the privacy of the home that the tremor quiets down.

Because of the tendency for symptoms to worsen during emotional pressure, some PD people consciously avoid all threatening social situations. Yet, while the hand may seem to the patient to be flopping around in a conspicuous and rowdy way, it is not especially obvious to others (who generally don't care very much anyway), and it actually oscillates at the relatively moderate rate of from 4 to 7 cycles per second. Compare this to the shaking produced by a benign essential tremor (see the next chapter) which, though it has a wide range of frequency, oscillates at rates of up to 20 cycles per second.

Lynn R., a member of a New York City Parkinson's group, found that whenever she and her husband visited friends she ended up spending much of the evening trying to keep her shaking leg out of sight. This battle was exhausting as well as embarrassing. She says:

> It's as if I have two big snakes down there that want to keep moving and wiggling around on their own. I found that whenever Greg and I saw friends and the conversation became animated, my legs would start to dance and move around. It becomes distracting. People pretend they don't see. But they do. Then I'd be half attentive to the conversation, half occupied with keeping my legs under control. Of course, I thought

everyone was staring at me and knew what I was trying to hide. So I just got silent during conversations for fear that if I talked too much I'd make my legs shake more.

Gradually, Lynn found that her enthusiasm for social occasions was outweighed by her fear of exposure. After a while she began encouraging her husband to attend these functions alone while she made limp excuses and spent the evening in front of the TV. In later chapters we will deal with these issues of fear and embarrassment so close to the heart of PD patients.

Rigidity

When medical professionals speak of *muscle tone* they refer to the degree to which a set of muscles can resist an applied force for a prolonged period of time; that is, the ability to resist an externally applied pressure such as a pulling or a pushing on the limb. In cases of Parkinson's disease, patients show a decided *increase* in muscle tone. This phenomenon is referred to as *rigidity*.

Rigidity is subjectively experienced as a feeling of stiffness and aching, especially in the major joints of the elbow, knee, and wrist. Technically speaking, these muscles are not stiff in the way they might be after a strenuous round of golf or tennis. They simply feel vaguely uncomfortable and, in fact, pain is often the earliest PD symptom to appear, especially joint pain.

Physicians in the examining room observe rigidity in a somewhat different way than the patient, as a slight but steady jerking movement felt when they passively manipulate a patient's arm or leg up and down, back and forth. This jerking motion produces a series of strangely regular, ratchet-like catches, as if the arm or leg was being raised and lowered on a set of slotted gears. For this reason, the increased muscular resistance common to PD is known as "cogwheel" rigidity: The movements have a cogwheel-like feel to them. When the limb behaves this way it is said to be "cogwheeling."

Almost all PD patients experience some degree of rigidity. It may manifest as an inability to move the elbows and ankles through the normal range of motion. Or it may reside in the hands, becoming troublesome to perform intricate motor activities such as sewing or writing a letter. Stiffness while walking is an especially common sign. It begins as a slight limp or drag in one leg, which is often unperceived on the part of the patient. Eventually the drag turns into a characteristic short-stepped gait that the nineteenth-century French doctor Jean-Martin Charcot described as *petit pas*—little steps—and which forces patients to take increasingly smaller and smaller strides as they move from point A to B, leaning forward as they go and involuntarily quickening their pace to a kind of mincing run. This feature is known as *festination* or *festinating gait* (from the Latin *festinare*, "to hasten") and ordinarily does not appear until both sides of the body are affected by rigidity.

Caregiver Hank K. talks about his wife:

At first she was stiff in the mornings. Then all during the day. Her fingers hurt at night. I told her she was dragging her leg. She didn't believe me. She'd look in the mirror and not see it. Later on she could see it. Today she has trouble getting started when she walks and is forced to take small paces which sometimes get out of control and she shoots across the room if there's no one around to catch her. I have seen her shoot ahead right into pieces of furniture.

Lawrence Van B., who developed PD in his late sixties, describes his first experience with rigidity:

I noticed it when I got up in the morning. My lower back and trunk hurt like hell and I hadn't done anything to antagonize them the day before. Then I apparently—I say apparently cause I didn't notice it myself—I started to hunch over as a result of these back pains, and my posture began to shift, became worse and more hunched. I'd wake up some mornings and my whole body felt stiff as a board. For no reason that I understood at the time. Had cramps in my legs which is something I'd never had. Just an overall feeling that I was hardening up and my limbs were getting tighter and harder on me. It was no fun, especially cause I couldn't figure out what was causing it.

Further Symptoms Caused by or Related to Rigidity

BENT OR ALTERED POSTURE.   PD people sometimes develop a
slightly bent, stooped posture. They tuck their chin into their chest
or incline their head forward. A slight but decided lean to one side
may occur. Those afflicted with such postural difficulties lose their
balance easily and fall (or sometimes backpeddle) at the slightest
provocation, a small misstep, say, or a brush against a scampering
cat or dog.

Bent posture, as far as it is understood, is a result of increased
muscle tone in the back and neck. In many cases it can be controlled by a combination of regular exercise and medication.

BENT ELBOWS AND ABDUCTED ARMS.   Like limping and foot
dragging, bent elbows and abducted arms, that is, arms turned out
and away from the body, are common early indications of Parkinson's. Victims carry their arms in a peculiar crooked, drawn-up
manner, sometimes with a hunch in the shoulders to match. As
with a limp, this change of posture may be noticed by family and
friends before the patient becomes aware of it:

Juanita O.: I didn't think anything was wrong until my
husband informed me that I was walking around with my arms
tucked up to my chest and kind of folded in at the shoulder
and elbow. It was involuntary. His remedy was for me to take
two heavy rocks and carry them around, one in each hand.
That didn't help much, needless to say. Friends suggested that
I had been moping around for a while, and also I taught
camping skills at Girl Scouts, and all of a sudden I was sitting
down on a rock and some of the girls would rush up to help
me when I started to stand up, and some of them wanted to
know why I was holding my arms in such weird positions. I
started wondering, Do they see something I don't? When my
tremor developed I went to a doctor and got started on the
Sinemet.

SPEECH DIFFICULTIES.   "It was just as if someone had turned
down my voice box volume" is the way one PD patient describes

it. "It was as if I was talking just as loud as before but people weren't hearing me as well. I thought the whole world was going deaf. Then people pointed out that my voice level was low."

It is estimated that approximately half the people suffering from Parkinson's disease develop speech disorders. The list of possible symptoms includes reduced voice volume, slurred or indistinct pronunciation, an inappropriately rapid (or sometimes slowed) rate of speech, poor modulation, uncontrolled repetition of words or phrases, plus several variations on these themes. Such complications are due to the rigidity of the lung and chest muscles that control inhalation and exhalation (and hence voice projection), plus the decreased efficiency of the muscle groups responsible for phonation and word articulation.

While anti-Parkinson's drugs control speech problems to some degree, another useful approach is to practice daily speech improvement exercises. These maneuvers include exercises that have been devised by speech therapists over the years and are targeted at specific problem areas such as amplification, pronunciation, speed of vocalization, facial expression, and breath control. A detailed sampling of these exercises will be described in a later chapter.

OVERALL SORENESS. Patients sometimes wake up in the morning feeling achy all over. Their back and joint muscles are painful, and these areas don't seem to loosen up easily as the morning moves on. Cramps may grip the calves and feet, especially after physical exercise. Chest tightening sometimes occurs, producing a gripping pain across the chest area not unlike angina. All such reactions can be a product of rigidity.

Slowness of Movement or Bradykinesia

For many years physicians believed that tremor and rigidity were the two major features of Parkinson's disease, and that bradykinesia-like behavior—extreme slowness of movement—was a kind of secondary reaction resulting from the two primary symptoms.

Exactly when bradykinesia was recognized as a third symptom

of PD is a debated issue. Some doctors claim that with the advent of stereotaxic surgery (see Chapter 10), whereby x-ray and electronic probes are used to apply pinpoint surgery to areas of a patient's brain, it became apparent that tremor and rigidity could be relieved but that the bradykinesia still remained, proving bradykinesia to be a discrete PD symptom unto itself. Other doctors, especially older neurologists, point out that even thirty years ago the importance of bradykinesia as a separate symptom of Parkinson's disease was being stressed in medical schools, and that through the decades a large number of neurologists have seen patients whose only PD symptom is bradykinesia.

Leaving such arguments to the medical historians, we can say here that bradykinesia, or *akinesia* as it is also called, is now fully recognized as a separate, definable, and highly problematic effect of Parkinson's disease that, though it is mild at the onset, tends to develop with inexorable relentlessness through the years until it often becomes the most debilitating of all complications. PD patients often complain of feeling weak or feeble, as if their limbs have become rubbery and the life is drained from them. This apparent weakness is a misperception. Objectively speaking, muscular force is not appreciably affected in the early stages of PD. Ask a PD person to squeeze your hand and their grip will be as firm as anyone's. What is actually taking place is that the muscles of Parkinson's sufferers are reacting less fluidly than before, and patients mistake this slowness and discomfort for lack of physical strength.

Yet another reason why bradykinesia is so problematic is that, unlike tremor, it is not a single symptom but a symptom complex. Following are the three chief components that typify it.

Delay in the Execution of Automatic Movements

Most of us swing our arms or tie our shoes as a matter of course. We don't think much about it. Yet with PD these movements are no longer a matter of routine. As one patient put it, "My body doesn't always do what I want it to anymore, so I have to keep telling it who's boss; where once my body did it all now my head has taken over."

The irony is that nothing is wrong with the PD person's motor system per se. The tendons, the nerves, and the muscles are intact. The problem stems from a breakdown in communication between the brain's commands for action and the body's response time in obeying them. In his usual precise way James Parkinson explains the phenomenon: "The muscles did not react normally to the dictates of the mind." "Parkinsonism disrupts the process at the very center where the orders for movement are formulated" writes Dr. K. A. Flowers, lecturer in psychology at the University of Hull, England. "The patient's difficulty stems from faulty instructions being sent [by the brain] to the motor system, rather than the motor system responding inaccurately."[2]

Observe PD patients when they are in the act of sitting down. They seem forced to *think about it*, to consciously consider how best to maneuver themselves into a sofa or chair. We can almost read their thoughts: "Now turn—stand by the side of the chair—grab the arms—hold tight—shift the weight—pivot the body—line up the backside with the cushion—bend the knees. . . ." The whole process is done in such a careful, methodical way that it appears to take place in slow motion.

Involuntary and quasi-involuntary movements are also affected by bradykinesia. PD people do not blink their eyes or swallow very often. They do not wrinkle their foreheads or mouths when they talk; they do not display the squints, face creasings, and eyebrow flexions that most of us make automatically during conversation. This immobility gives the face a fixed, glacial appearance, well known as the *Parkinson's mask*. Nor are the anticipated shifts of the eyes and head apparent. The person's eyes may bulge, causing the pupils to appear dry and red, adding further to the strangeness of the picture. This again is bradykinesia.

It is interesting to consider the extent to which we take such anatomical movements for granted; we notice them only in their absence. How interesting as well that seemingly minor facial movements turn out to be decisive cues in the communication of feelings and intentions, and that when these subliminal signals are absent confusion and misunderstanding result. Because of their facial immobility PD people appear to be unresponsive and indifferent, even sullen. In fact, they are sitting on a mountain of unexpressed thoughts, moods, and emotions. Caregivers and family alike would do well to keep this fact in mind and not take undemonstrativeness as a sign of disinterest.

Inability to Shift Easily from One Motor Pattern to Another

If a Parkinsonian patient is walking across a room and someone suddenly asks him or her to stop, turn around, walk to the left, and pick up an object from the floor, the person will often become disoriented and may be forced to take a number of small, hesitating steps before getting onto the new track. Here bradykinesia interferes with the ability to make quick, sudden changes in direction and to execute more than one activity at a time.

Molly R., a Parkinson patient for seven years, can stir batter in a bowl without difficulty. If someone asks her to pick up a pan and stir at the same time, however, she gets flustered. Molly has to pause, get her bearings, put the spoon down carefully, and concentrate fully on the pan. *Then* she can accomplish the task, but only after directing all her attention to this single activity.

As Dr. Andre Barbeau, a well-known expert on neurological diseases, explains, the PD person tends to act "as if at any one time he is capable of conceptualizing and generating only a single plan or program. Any change requires the interpretation of feedback data and the reformulation of both strategy and tactics, with the inherent time lag being considerably increased, every movement having to be 'thought out' in detail."[3]

Bouts of Intense Fatigue

Mary G. speaks of her early Parkinson's onset:

I was a fifty-three-year-old woman and very energetic. Very. I worked as a secretary in a commercial glass firm. One day—it seemed overnight but they tell me it's supposed to take longer—everything started being such a chore for things. Every time my boss asked me to get such-and-such a record it seemed I was down in the files for hours. Hours! My hands weren't working right, you know, as if they weren't my usual hands. But worst of all was that I got so *tired!* So easily. I'd get up to walk to the conference room, walk back, and have to rest. This was unheard of for me. I didn't know what was going on.

Sudden fatigue is a major feature of bradykinesia and affects at least 80 to 90 percent of patients. Its onset is unpredictable, like many other parkinsonian symptoms, arriving out of the blue and leaving just as quickly. For some people, frequent rests are the necessary antidote. For others, becoming familiar with one's good times and bad times of day and planning accordingly is the key.

Other Symptoms Caused by or Related to Bradykinesia

DISTURBED GAIT. A change in gait is a common early indicator of PD, especially when people develop a slight drag in their leg or begin to limp for no apparent reason. Two members of a Parkinson's group speak on the subject:

Jose M.: Kathy (my wife) started telling me I was limping one day. I was not aware of it but then it got a little worse. That's how it started. It was a very slow drag, as if I was pulling my foot along behind me sort of, but I wasn't aware I was doing it. Slight but not slight enough for people not to notice, enough for my wife to get me to a neurologist.

Leslie de V.: My husband was working overseas and I was at home. I noticed that my right foot was dragging a bit. But I had tripped at one time and I thought it was due to the tripping. Then my daughter and I went on a trip to Greece. At Mikanos my daughter and I found a building we wanted to see at the top of the hill. We couldn't get there by taxi so we had to walk. I started to notice that I had trouble walking up the hill. My foot was really dragging and my feet weren't doing what they were supposed to do. That was the real beginning of things. But it wasn't till some years later that I actually got a diagnosis.

FESTINATING GAIT. A related problem occurs when patients have difficulty walking and are forced to take a series of short, mincing steps to establish forward momentum. A kind of shuffle, really, these steps are inappropriately short at first, then become proportionately quicker until they turn into choppy strides. One patient dubbed it the "Charlie Chaplin strut."

Related both to rigidity and bradykinesia, when a person with festinating gait moves forward it is medically known as *propulsive gait* (though PD people refer to it more idiomatically as the "car-without-brakes" syndrome). When the movement is backward or back-peddling it is called *retropulsive gait.* When the movement is sideways it is called *lateral gait.*

IMPAIRED BALANCE. Although severe balance disorders ordinarily come after Parkinson's has progressed for many years, random falls can take place at any time, and patients must be on the alert to avoid positioning themselves in precarious postures. Such episodes seem unprovoked. Patients simply lose their footing and tumble to the ground—they weren't pushed and they didn't trip.

Matty (Nick B.'s wife): Before Nick retired I noticed he was getting different. In 1975, the year I learned to ride a bike, we were biking all over the place together. Nick was an expert, could ride without hands, that kind of thing. But the following year we would be riding along and suddenly he'd just fall off his bike for no reason, like one of those episodes in a comedy movie. He couldn't keep his balance anymore. We went from doctor to doctor for almost ten years to find out what was wrong. They diagnosed it as nerve damage because Nick has diabetes. Finally, when some of the other symptoms appeared, we realized what the problem really was.

Mike A.: I retired at age sixty-five. I didn't have a stroke or anything like that. But I started to lose my balance in walking. I was diagnosed as Parkinson's. When I look back I can see it was coming gradually all along. I used to like to dance with my wife. We'd take dancing lessons, but suddenly I couldn't keep up with her anymore on the dance floor. The slowness. And sometimes I'd just take a fall or slip back when we were dancing and she'd have to grab me. It happened over about a five-year time period. When you look backward you can see the progress of a thing better, how it advanced without you really knowing it was there.

SWALLOWING DIFFICULTIES. The throat muscles, similar to the muscles that control breathing and speech, lose their contractive strength and coordination in parkinsonism. This slowdown affects the finely tuned muscles of the larynx, which no longer rise and fall automatically, and the epiglottis, which now fails to fold back in its normal way. Not only is the saliva-swallowing process affected but people tend to develop chewing difficulties, food residue buildup in the mouth, digestive disorders, and, most troublesome, choking.

These complications, alarming as they seem at first, are usually controllable, but only if patients make conscious attempts to develop new eating and swallowing habits. Suggestions are in Chapter 13.

A related problem that also stems from swallowing disturbance is excessive saliva buildup. Drooling is a messy nuisance as well as a social embarrassment. It can irritate the throat and palate, inviting rawness and bacterial infection. While some anti-Parkinson's drugs automatically reduce saliva buildup, especially the antihistamine and anticholinergic drugs, learned voluntary control of swallowing may also be necessary if the problem is to be kept under control. Help along these lines is given in Chapter 13.

MICROGRAPHIA. Odd as it seems, sudden changes in the size of handwriting, a condition known medically as *micrographia,* can be one of the earliest indications of PD. It is characterized by a strangely unsteady sensation in the writing hand, with penmanship becoming accordingly affected and words appearing atypically shaky and small.

Particularly characteristic is a handwriting that begins normal-sized, then becomes progressively smaller as it runs across the page. A person reading such a sample might suppose the writer is intentionally trying to reduce the size of the words from the beginning of the line to the end. However, PD people are often unaware of the degree to which their penmanship is declining. Altered handwriting is a common early indication of PD and is often the symptom that sends people to a physician. It is not entirely clear if it occurs from rigidity or bradykinesia, or both. As with many symptoms, it becomes difficult at a certain point to distinguish between the two causes.

CHANGE IN BOWEL AND/OR URINARY HABITS. Typical of PD to varying degrees is constipation, urinary incontinence, and difficulty in urinating. Medications sometimes make matters worse.

While constipation is often discussed at self-help groups, among friends, or with a physician, urinary incontinence is something of a taboo and may continue to harass sufferers for years before the matter is aired with a professional. Neither condition should be ignored or minimized.

EYE PROBLEMS. Since the mechanism that causes the eyelids to open and close is adversely affected by PD, patients frequently go long periods of time without blinking. Blinking is, of course, a reflex mechanism designed to protect, clean, and moisturize the eye area, and the lack of it causes the soft areas around the eyes to become dry and red, causing bloodshot pupils or, more seriously, conjunctivitis, an inflammation of the mucus membranes that line the eye. In a few instances, people will suffer from an inability to open (or keep open) their eyelids at all, a condition known medically as *blepharospasm*.

To prevent bloodshot eyes and conjunctivitis, hygiene and daily eye care are usually sufficient. Blepharospasm, which is sometimes caused by the anti-Parkinson's drugs themselves, is more complicated and is best dealt with by a physician.

BREATHING DIFFICULTIES. PD people often become easily winded or have difficulty catching their breath. Assuming that this condition does not stem from heart or lung disease (in which case a considerably different medical approach must obviously be taken), labored breathing traces back to one of two problems.

The first is rigidity and/or bradykinesia, which affects the lung muscles and exerts a restricting influence on the expansion of the chest wall. In this case, medication ordinarily sets the problem straight. The second possibility is that the medications themselves are restricting the breathing. Reduction or modification of drug dose is usually the answer.

BUT YOU NEVER KNOW

The symptom list so far is representative though by no means inclusive. Other symptoms will come, perhaps, though which ones no one can say for sure. PD patients may experience depression, sleep disturbance, swollen feet, conjunctivitis, nausea, stomach-ache, fatigue, excessive sweating, skin problems—or they may not. It depends on the individual, the medications, and the degree to which the disease has developed.

Whatever you do, therefore, don't assume that since you have had Parkinson's for two years now, or four years, or seven, that you should be experiencing X, Y, or Z symptoms. PD doesn't work this way, and there is a good chance that if a particular symptom has not bothered you up till now it will not bother you at all.

Although many of the characteristic complaints of PD are uncomfortable and at times distressing, in most cases there is some kind of remedial option available to make them tolerable. In Part III we will examine these options in detail. Don't assume that because a handicap is persistent it can't be controlled. Help is out there, sometimes closer than you think. You simply have to know where—and how—to find it.

NOTES

1. Roger Duvoisin, M.D., *Parkinson's Disease: A Guide for Patient and Family* (New York: Raven Press, 1984), 16–17.

2. Richard L. Gregory, ed., *The Oxford Companion to the Mind* (New York: Oxford University Press, 1987), 588.
3. Andre Barbeau, "Parkinson's Disease: Clinical Features and Etiopathology." In Vinken, P., Bruyn, G., and Klawans, H., eds., *Handbook of Clinical Neurology,* vol. 5 (New York: Elsevier Science Publishers, 1986), 92.

3

At the Doctor's Office: Examination, Diagnosis, and Prognosis

Although no single test exists to definitively determine if a person does or does not have Parkinson's disease, recognizing PD is, all things considered, a relatively cut-and-dry task in most instances. However, there are pitfalls that may trap even the most seasoned practitioner.

To begin, there are not one but several kinds of Parkinson's disease. The type we are concerned with is known as *ideopathic Parkinson's,* that is, "of unknown origin." This is the common variety, and the kind most frequently seen in the examining room. Other forms exist as well: some temporary, some permanent, some induced by drugs, and some induced by pollutants, toxic chemicals, or even a species of influenza. All require careful testing and observation on the part of the examining physician to tell them apart.

To complicate matters, many other diseases are characterized by symptoms that are similar to those of PD. Tremor is probably the most conspicuous of these look-alike symptoms, although there is a range of other possibilities including fatigue, stiffness, joint pain, and postural changes. More than one person suffering from early PD has, in fact, been sent home from the doctor's office with a supposed clean bill of health, informed that stress is the real problem, or that the person's symptoms are merely the result of increasing age.

Despite these and several other points at which a diagnosis can go awry, specialists have the advantage of being able to base their diagnosis on characteristic symptoms that are, by and large, common to Parkinson's disease and to no other: A PD tremor is different from the tremor of palsy or hyperthyroidism or alcoholism; cogwheel rigidity is a different kind of rigidity than that of arthritis or Wilson's disease; and so forth.

What can a person with possible PD involvement expect from an initial exam visit? What signs and symptoms will the doctor be looking for? What type of exam will be administered, what tests will be called for, and how long will it take before the diagnosis is reached? And what then?

AT THE DOCTOR'S OFFICE

A neurological examination of any kind is, broadly speaking, composed of four discrete, though overlapping, diagnostic parts. These are:

1. An *observation* of the patient's overall appearance and behavior including movement, posture, gesture, speech, and mood
2. An *interview* designed to determine a person's medical and personal history
3. A *neurological exam* with appropriate tests, if needed, plus a thorough physical exam
4. A *mental status exam*

Observation of the Patient

The first, most direct, and perhaps most effective method of diagnosing PD is by simple observation and intuitive assessment of a person's overall appearance and behavior. People with PD often display behavioral quirks that are patently characteristic of parkinsonism, and a trained physician will pick them up in the first few minutes of the examination.

Tremor, for instance, especially a slow tremor located in the hand or foot, is an obvious clue. This, conjoined with slowness of movement, say, or speech problems, or postural abnormality such as a crooked arm, are all flags that cause physicians to consider a Parkinson's diagnosis. Further tests will of course be made.

Jon Dorman, M.D., a neurologist in private practice in Danville, Virginia, says:

> If the truth be told, the diagnosis for Parkinson's disease is often made at a glance. It's often obvious. Parkinsonism reduces a person's motor activity, the frequency of their facial expressions, their movement in general. Walking is slower. Less stable. The person loses balance easily. He is sometimes bent over. There is a new and overall kind of ploddingness that was not there before. There really aren't a whole lot of other diseases that affect a person quite this way, unless, of course, it's a neurological disorder that has a form of parkinsonism associated with it. So when a possible PD patient comes into my office I just observe their movements as they walk across the room, or as they get in and out of a chair, or climb onto the examination table. If I see Parkinson's-like signs then I assess the rest of the clinical picture, rule out other possibilities, and come to a conclusion. The physical and mental exams that follow usually just help me confirm what I've already suspected from the very start.

Robert Barrett, M.D., a neurologist in private practice in New York City, adds to these observations:

> In old-time medicine, doctors were trained to diagnose from sight as much as by equipment. Today machines have more or less taken over the diagnostic job, though with Parkinson's disease there is still a place for simple observation. When a patient comes into my examination

room I ask her to walk across the room for me. I ask her a few telling questions. I watch the way she moves and interacts with the physical world. This tells me a lot. A whole lot. The rest is often just confirmation.

The Patient's Medical and Personal History

Parkinson's disease is such a slow, insidious ailment that patients tend not to pay much attention to its symptoms at first, and if they do, they may dismiss them as quirks of aging. It thus becomes the physician's job to recognize these early symptoms and to help patients identify them. One of the most effective methods is taking the personal/medical history.

While the questions that may be asked at such a session are legion, a prudent physician will tailor the inquiry to the patient's needs and condition. A sample of possible questions at the first visit (and that should be considered before this visit takes place) includes the following:

- When did you first notice your symptoms? Describe them in detail.
- What was the first thing you noticed about them? What were you doing at the time?
- In what ways and at what rate have the symptoms progressed?
- Was, or is, there any pain involved? Describe it.
- In what ways do you find that your health has changed over the past six to twelve months?

Thorough physicians will inquire about seemingly unrelated medical issues:

- How has your general health been through the years? Did you have any major physical problems as a child or as a young person?
- What type of operations or chronic disorders have you experienced during your lifetime?

- Do you suffer from allergies? Are you allergic to specific medications? Which ones?
- Do you exercise? When, and how frequently?
- Describe your general diet.
- Do you have sleep problems?
- Do neurological diseases run in your family? Which ones?

Since certain forms of parkinsonism are caused by toxic substances, doctors will want to know about the person's occupation and domestic environment:

- What is your occupation, where do you work, and how long have you been employed in this position?
- Does (or did) your job bring you into contact with chemicals or toxic wastes? Which ones?
- Have you been exposed to large amounts of carbon monoxide or toxic gases during the past few years?
- Is your home located near a factory or a processing plant?
- Do you have hobbies that require the use of glues, dyes, petroleum-based sprays, and so forth?

Certain forms of Parkinson's disease are encephalitis-related:

- Have you ever suffered from any form of encephalitis?
- Describe any major childhood diseases.
- Did you ever suffer from a particularly serious form of flu as a young person? Describe it.

Physical traumas will be discussed:

- Have you recently been in an accident or undergone a head trauma?
- Did you receive any major head injury as a child or as a young person?
- What type of contact sports have you indulged in over the years?

Psychological modalities are important:

- Have you recently experienced a severe psychological or emotional shock? Has a loved one recently died? Have you recently lost a job?
- Are you depressed? Do you have a history of chronic depression?

General state of health and recent physical complaints will be profiled:

- How is your appetite? Do your bowels move regularly? Do you have any digestion problems?
- Do you smoke? If so, for how long and how many cigarettes each day?
- Do you drink? If so, for how long and how much do you consume each day?
- How is your everyday energy level?
- Have you had any recent surgery?
- Are you presently suffering from any type of chronic disorder, either physical or mental?
- How would you describe your state of health in general?

Many of these questions have little to do directly with Parkinson's disease, yet when considered as a whole they give examining physicians a three-dimensional portrait of the person, a kind of bird's eye view of who they are and how they tick. That's important. Dr. Barrett says:

The most significant thing you can do for a Parkinson's patient is to spend time taking a medical and personal history. It has to be documented if you're going to get a total picture and deal with the person as a whole person. I like to know things such as was there anything wrong with their birth? Was it prolonged? Was it a toxic birth? Did their mother have difficulty carrying them? What has life been like in general? Where have they lived most of their life? What kind of infectious diseases have they had? Have they ever been jaundiced? What kinds of diseases run in their family?

I don't know what this has to do with things, really, but in my records it gives me bits of information, threads that I can follow throughout a person's life. For instance, I have a patient who developed Parkinson's disease at age sixty-five. He's a psychiatrist who lives in an old Victorian house in Orange County where he sees his patients. This man tells me that for years people have been coming into his office and saying they smell gas. Finally, he had the gas lines checked and, sure enough, leaks were found. So I started wondering: Was there a relationship between this man's condition and the many years he spent inhaling the gas? Perhaps there was. Perhaps, I told myself, I should pay more attention to this line of reasoning.

Then there's another patient I've followed for years who has developed rigid hypokinetic parkinsonism. Some time ago he and his wife went camping for a week in a cabin in Maine. It was the middle of the winter and they were using a propane stove to keep warm. One night they fell asleep and the gas escaped from the stove. The man woke up, dragged himself and his wife through the door, but by the time they got outside she was already dead. The man then spent a long period of time in the hospital recovering. Now propane gas poisoning causes hypoxic changes in the brain, and it is a well-known fact that carbon monoxide can produce a clinical syndrome that looks like Parkinson's. Today this fellow stoops, shuffles, has a slight tremor, suffers from obvious bradykinesia. In other words, he has what appears to be Parkinson's disease. Was his condition caused by the gas? I'm not sure. But if I hadn't found out about this experience I would certainly have had a lot less data to go by when I diagnosed him.

A Thorough General and Neurological Examination with Appropriate Tests, When Needed

A thorough physical exam is given including blood and urine sampling, measurement of cholesterol levels, and checking of the heart and lungs. Once the person's overall health is established, a series of neurological tests will be made. Although doctors vary somewhat in their choice of diagnostic routines, the procedures discussed below are standard.

Checking for Tremor

Since PD patients do not always demonstrate their full range of symptoms during the short period of time in which they are in the examining room, simple diagnostic tricks may be necessary to elicit them. While the examiner is chatting informally with the patient he or she will be carefully watching the patient for signs of tremor. More overtly, doctors sometimes place a sheet of paper over a patient's hands and check for vibrating movements. Some doctors ask patients to hold their arms in front of them with their eyes closed. Patients may be asked to draw simple designs and these will be examined for any telltale line unsteadiness. Doctors may ask patients to fill out medical forms that are then studied for micrographia.

Since a tremor tends to increase when patients are nervous, and since doctors' offices are notoriously anxiety-provoking places, a PD tremor will usually become more and more conspicuous as the examination goes on.

Testing Muscle Tone and Rigidity

Tone or tonicity, as described in Chapter 2, is measured by a muscle's ability to resist an applied external force. When parkinsonism is present tonicity will be dramatically increased, with a resultant increase in rigidity. Examining physicians test a person's arms or legs for this reaction, and if it is observed, along with a tremor, the combination makes it fairly certain that parkinsonism is present.

One of the initial tests doctors perform during an exam is to push, pull, or otherwise manipulate a patient's arms and legs in an effort to find cogwheeling or the more uniform but equally typical muscular resistance known as "lead-pipe" rigidity. One particular maneuver, the so-called *Noika-Froment*, requires that the patient's wrist be moved until it becomes entirely passive. The patient is then asked to slowly raise his or her other arm while continuing to move the wrist. If rigidity is present, an almost instantaneous increase in muscle tone will be apparent to both doctor and patient.

Dr. Jon Dorman says:

If I asked a normal person to lie down and totally relax and give me no resistance whatsoever, and if I picked his arm up, it would be floppy, like a ragdoll. With Parkinson's disease a patient's arm tends to be more stiff. If you move the joints back and forth they never seem really to relax. Instead you feel a catching, slotted movement as you manipulate them—bup, bup, bup, like a rachet. Cogwheeling. This cogwheeling is, in effect, related to the tremor. It's picking up the tremor through the passive movement of the patient's limb.

Rigidity can also be measured by direct observation. A doctor will request that patients walk across the room, and will then note that their arms hang passively at their side, or that shuffling or tiptoe walking is apparent, which possibly indicates PD. Patients may be asked to draw a series of spirals; when studied these designs may appear small and cramped. Sometimes doctors ask patients to write several sentences and then examine the script for squiggly lines, for deficits in the loops of the "Y" and "J", and for illegibility or inappropriately small letters, which are signs that rigidity has developed in the intricately balanced alternating motions of the hand muscles.

Much can be deduced from conversation. A physician notices when a patient's voice level is unnaturally low, a possible sign of increased muscle tone in the voice box and vocal chords. Or doctors may ask a patient covert diagnostic questions. The interview could go something like this:

DOCTOR: Are you having difficulty getting in and out of the front seat of your car these days? Trouble sliding over laterally?

PATIENT: Matter of fact, I am.

DOCTOR: And when you walk into a closet or small space you sometimes find it's hard to turn around?

PATIENT: How did you know that?

DOCTOR: Let me also suggest that you have occasional problems pulling your coat or dress up and over your head?

PATIENT: Definitely.

DOCTOR: That it's hard for you to turn from side to side when you're in bed. That sometimes people ask you to repeat yourself. Or they tell you that you're not speaking loudly enough.

PATIENT: Yes to all of these, Doctor. You must be a mind reader!

But the doctor is not a mind reader. He simply knows that these patterns of behavior are all related in one way or another to the insidious onset of rigidity, tremor, and bradykinesia.

Testing for Bradykinesia

Bradykinesia is most effectively determined by testing a person's ability to make quick, alternating movements. Patients are directed to tap their fingers against their thumbs in rapid succession. People with Parkinson's will perform the first several taps without difficulty; then on the third or fourth attempt their fingers will tend to "stick" or to freeze.

Similar diagnostic exercises call for tapping cadences with the fingers or feet, opening and closing the hands in rapid succession, alternately raising and lowering the heel and toes of one foot. If these movements are jerky, irregular, interrupted, or if they decrease in size and energy as they continue, there is reason to suspect bradykinesia. Patients may also be asked to draw clockwise circles with the right and left hands simultaneously. Oddly enough, PD people are able to sketch opposite turning circles far more easily than circles that turn in the same direction.

More directly, examinees are asked to sit on a sofa for a quarter of an hour and are then told to stand up quickly. People with PD often need to rock back and forth several times before they can get to their feet. In other situations patients are given several minutes to put together a picture puzzle and their times are then checked against a statistical norm. If the score is low, and if a patient's hands seemed clumsy and slow while assembling the pieces, this is a further indication that bradykinesia is at work.

Testing Reflex and Sensory Status

Whereas some PD people show hyperactive reflexes, others present sluggish reflexes that seem lacking in pep and bounce. Either condition is possible with Parkinson's. Most frequently, though, PD people demonstrate relatively normal reflexes, and those who test poorly in this area often have secondary neurological problems along with the Parkinson's.

The *Babinski* (or *flexor plantar reflex*) is one of the best known of the reflex tests. The doctor rubs the sole of the patient's foot with a reflex hammer and watches for a downward inflection of the toe. If the toe goes up rather than down, this may indicate a nerve irregularity. As a general rule, PD people test normally for the Babinski, and if the results are abnormal, secondary involvements such as a tumor or stroke may be considered.

Also tested is the ability to perceive pain, touch, vibration, and position. Doctors will trace a number on the patient's hand and tell them to describe it. Or they will hand patients a common object like a key or a pencil and ask them to identify it with their eyes closed. Though PD people often have stiff hands and poor finger control, they generally do well in such sensory exams and can easily identify an object by its shape, texture, size, and temperature.

Testing for Postural Stability

A standard test for postural stability calls for the patient to stand erect with eyes open. The examiner places one hand on the patient's back and delivers a light push to the chest with the other. People with parkinsonism tend to step back stiffly when handled this way, sometimes without making any attempt to regain their balance. They may, in fact, propel to the rear so quickly that the physician is forced to catch them from falling.

Other postural stability tests call for patients to close their eyes, extend their arms in front of them, and hold this position while they are observed. They may be asked to stand on one foot and then the other, to sit in a chair and stand up again, or to simply walk around the room.

Other tests

A variety of other tests and observations may be conducted. Doctors will examine ocular movements and reflexes. They will check hearing and draw blood samples. The cranial nerves may be examined through the eyes and, if appropriate, a CAT (computerized axial tomography) scan or x-ray will be ordered. The joints are usually looked at along with the muscles and ligaments. Pulses are taken, the heart is listened to, and an EEG (electroencephalogram) is ordered. The possibilities are varied and are usually tailored to a person's particular age, condition, and symptoms.

Mental Status Exam

In medical school students are taught to determine a patient's mental status by posing questions of orientation regarding time, place, and person. However, asking intelligent, with-it patients their name, telephone number, and the day of the week can be as insulting to the examinee as it is embarrassing for the physician. Rather than administer such formal mental status exams, most mental testing for PD is done on an informal, even invisible way.

Some physicians, for instance, test for dementia by initiating a casual discussion with the patient on current affairs. Others take a patient's personal history and in so doing ask questions that determine general levels of awareness. Still others ask patients to perform simple mathematical calculations, ostensibly as part of the physical exam (physicians may have a patient count to 30 by 3's while standing on one foot). If cognitive deficits exist they will reveal themselves during these tests.

Generally speaking, dementia is not a major issue in the early stages of PD, and for many years physicians did not believe that intelligence, reason, or memory were affected by it at all. Today, due to improved medications, PD patients live longer than before and it is now recognized that memory and speed of thought are both diminished to some extent over time, but often in a mild way, and usually not until the disease has progressed considerably.

TYPES OF PARKINSONISM

While a majority of people diagnosed with PD have ideopathic Parkinson's, other forms exist, most of them unusual. Here the diagnostic going can get tough, especially when a person has, for example, a combination of Alzheimer's disease and Parkinson's, or Parkinson's-like symptoms that cannot be diagnosed as ideopathic Parkinson's.

Rather than wander in these complex and uncertain diagnostic labyrinths, let us briefly review the possible types of parkinsonism that a doctor may see in the examining room, have a look at the stages of symptom development that Parkinson's follows, and then move on to the more critical concerns of medication, self-help, and symptom relief.

Postencephalitic Parkinson's

In 1916 a flu epidemic appeared in various parts of the United States, causing symptoms that were dangerously similar to those of encephalitis. This scourge raged on for several years, damaging the basal ganglia area in the brain of patients and leaving a trail of paralysis and insanity in its wake. Approximately half the people who contracted the disease died, while survivors were left with severe mental and physical handicaps. The epidemic tapered off in the mid-1920s and died out entirely in the next decade; but its effects would return to haunt its victims.

For, as it turned out, almost everyone who experienced this ailment soon began to develop progressive, Parkinson's-like complications that were due, apparently, to the effect of the virus. Symptoms included rigidity, slowness, lethargy, involuntary movements of the eyes (which rolled upward in the head and remained "stuck" in this position for long periods of time), and bizarre mental changes.

Although the causes of the flu and its possible relationship to Parkinson's disease have been studied assiduously by medical researchers since this time, a great deal of confusion still surrounds this mysterious epidemic. Fortunately, it now seems to have disappeared from the population entirely, and today only a handful of parkinsonians are alive who can trace their condition back to the terrible event. As far as present studies indicate, new cases of postencephalitic Parkinson's are rare, and despite the Parkinson's-like effects that the flu produced in its sufferers, there is no convincing evidence to show that ideopathic Parkinson's disease itself is in any way triggered by a virus.

Drug–Related Parkinsonism

Certain medicinal drugs, we now know, block the action of dopamine in the brain and induce temporary Parkinson's-like reactions. Neuroleptic drugs are the most typical culprits, especially the more powerful tranquilizers in the chlorpromazine family such as *Thorazine* (known in Europe as *Largactil*), *Stelazine,* and *Prolixin.* A closely related drug, *Haldol,* is particularly likely to produce these reactions, while *Reserpine,* a blood pressure medication, can occasionally induce Parkinson's-like effects when taken in high doses.

However, only a few patients are adversely affected by these drugs, and less potent tranquilizers are available that rarely produce reactions such as *Valium, Librium,* and *Xanax.* The Parkinson's-like complaints that these drugs do cause are usually transient and temporary—but not always. In some cases it is known that they produce forms of parkinsonism that do not go away.

Environmental Triggers

Manganese and carbon monoxide poisoning are known to bring about damaging changes to the dopamine-producing parts of the brain and are capable of producing PD-like debilities such as tremor, rigidity, loss of muscle movement, and a tendency to walk on the tiptoes (a condition known clinically as *demarche de coq*).

Such reactions are brought on by local toxic conditions. Mine workers, for instance, occasionally develop PD-like symptoms after handling manganese ore for many years. Welders or workers in chemical plants can show similar symptoms following long-term exposure to manganese-laden chemicals; so can failed car-exhaust suicides who have managed to inhale massive amounts of carbon monoxide during their attempts.

Though the afflictions produced by these poisonous contacts are Parkinson's-like, they do not necessarily mimic ideopathic Parkinson's per se and they tend to be readily diagnosable, especially if the medical history shows that the patient has handled a specific contaminant for many years. Moreover, unless doctors specialize in industrially produced neurological diseases, they are unlikely to see more than one or two such cases during their entire careers.

Head Trauma

The medical case of Muhammad Ali received a great deal of press several years ago and inspired considerable speculation concerning the relationship between head trauma and Parkinson's disease. Muhammad Ali was, of course, the embattled and longtime world boxing champion who, despite a number of remarkable early matches in which his great skill allowed him to avoid being hit in the head at all, ended his career taking a number of terrible head poundings in some of the fiercest ring encounters of modern times. After his retirement, Ali promptly developed a PD-like syndrome, and this sad situation caused professionals and laypeople to wonder if repeated blows to the head do not in some as-yet unexplained way produce parkinsonism.

There are, it is true, a multitude of anecdotal cases telling of people who have been punched in the head, kicked in the eye, or thrown forward in an auto accident who soon afterward developed parkinsonism. Does this necessarily mean that Parkinson's disease and head trauma are related? Investigations have been going on for some time now and the verdict remains unclear. In many cases, the stories about head injuries and PD are clearly coincidence or hearsay. And as far as researchers have been able to determine, prize fighters, football players, practitioners of the martial arts, and those who receive repeated shocks to the head as part of their occupation (such as a jackhammer operator) experience no higher incidence of PD than do members of the general population.

At the same time, it is theoretically feasible that head trauma does damage the pathways running from the substantia nigra to the striatum, or that some as-yet unknown alterations take place when the brain is continually shaken. It is also a possibility that head traumas trigger a parkinsonian tendency that has long been present in an incipient state. There are many theories.

MPTP

It is not unusual for an important discovery in medical science to occur as a by-product of a seemingly unrelated event. In this instance, the development of the new and highly touted Parkinson's drug, Deprenyl, came about due to the baleful shenanigans of a group of California narcotic drug manufacturers.

As the story goes, several renegade chemists in San Jose put their heads together one day to invent a new designer drug that they hoped would mimic the effects of Demerol, and that could be produced cheaply and sold in quantity. Due to critical miscalculations in the laboratory, instead of producing Demerol the befuddled chemists manufactured a similar compound known as MPTP—methyl phenyl tetrahydropyridine.

Vending this substance as the latest in inexpensive highs, it soon turned out that anyone unlucky enough to inject it quickly developed severe and permanent Parkinson's-like symptoms, complete with typical 3- to 7-cycle tremor, muscular rigidity, and bradykinesia. Victims even responded to L-dopa and other PD medications in much the same way as parkinsonians do. Fortunately, only a handful of people took the MPTP before it was cleaned off the streets. Those who did take it—mostly young people—remain crippled with parkinsonism, probably for life.

News of this bizarre and tragic event spread quickly across the country and into various circles of the scientific community where investigations indicated that MPTP's tendency to create parkinsonism might be harnessed to a positive purpose—that under laboratory conditions it could be used to induce an experimental model of Parkinson's disease in laboratory animals.

Tests were conducted and researchers learned that when animals were given a drug called Deprenyl and then injected with MPTP they became immune to MPTP's toxic effects. A nationwide study of Parkinson's disease was subsequently launched known as DATA TOP, and eventually it became evident that Deprenyl boosts dopamine production in the brain and that many PD patients indeed improve with its use. Ironically, this discovery might never have been made if a handful of young addicts had not taken MPTP in the first place. Happily, MPTP poisoning among drug users seems to have been limited to the particular incident in San Jose, and few if any similar cases have been reported since then. Deprenyl is discussed in Chapter 9.

PARKINSON'S DISEASE LOOK-ALIKES

Besides the varieties of PD discussed so far, there are several other disorders and symptom syndromes that, though produced by separate causes and not related to Parkinson's disease per se, produce symptoms that resemble PD closely enough to be confusing and sometimes even confounding to the examining physician. These look-alike disorders include the following:

Aftermath of Stroke

Since the part of the brain that is frequently affected by stroke controls balance and forward gait, stroke victims sometimes present symptoms that resemble those of PD. People so afflicted may walk with a slow gait, jumble their words, or appear bent and unsteady on their feet. When L-dopa or a similarly effective medication is prescribed, it produces little or no improvement. This fact, coupled with the knowledge that the patient has had a major stroke (or a series of small ones) and that other symptoms not common to PD are present, is a tip-off that the condition arises from the stroke alone and not from Parkinson's involvement.

Brain Tumor

When performing a neurological exam, doctors often ask for a CAT scan, x-ray, or some type of nuclear magnetic resonance imaging (MRI) test. Occasionally patients or family members complain about this request, claiming that physicians order tests without substantial reason, and that since the brain changes brought about by PD cannot be detected by a CAT scan or x-ray, these high-technology, high-cost tests are a waste of time.

Such complaints notwithstanding, there is sound logic behind ordering these procedures. Since certain tumors produce Parkinson's-like symptoms, especially those located near the substantia nigra or the striatum, physicians order CAT scans and x-rays on the chance that the symptoms are due to such a growth, and to pinpoint the areas of the brain where it may be forming. If such suspicions are prevalent, this extra bit of precaution is certainly not out of line. Early detection of a tumor can prove to be nine-tenths of the cure.

Progressive Supranuclear Palsy

The hallmark symptom of supranuclear palsy is an impairment of the voluntary motor control of the eye movements that renders patients incapable of vertically elevating or lowering their gaze. A commonly reported early sign occurs when patients are unable to focus their eyes on their feet as they descend a flight of stairs.

Since this complaint is unlike anything experienced in parkinsonism, physicians who see patients with rigidity and gait disturbances coupled with poor voluntary control of vertical gaze will immediately suspect progressive supranuclear palsy. Other tip-offs include an early onset of dementia (memory loss coupled with inappropriate emotional behavior), rigidity in the neck and lower back instead of in the extremities, and a fluid type of rigidity unlike the typical PD cogwheel effect. Whereas PD people characteristically display a simianlike posture with a forward stoop and chin weighted toward the chest, progressive supranuclear palsy sufferers walk with their head hyperextended and the trunk tilted forward. The cause and cure for this disease are unknown.

Shy–Drager Syndrome

Known also as *primary orthostatic hypotension,* people suffering from this rare, progressive nerve disease display a mild PD syndrome along with bowel dysfunction, impotence, breathing problems, lack of tone in the bladder, and other indications of deranged functioning involving the autonomic nervous system. The characteristic that distinguishes it most clearly from Parkinson's disease is an inability to maintain normal blood pressure when in an upright position: Some patients actually lose consciousness when they try to stand up.

Essential Tremor

Also known as benign hereditary tremor, essential tremors are located in the hands, head, or even the voice. Generally they oscillate faster than the Parkinson's tremor and move through a wider range of variations.

Benign tremor, contrary to opinion, is not exclusive to the elderly and can even appear in adolescents. Its cause is believed to be hereditary. Voluntary movement and extreme emotions increase shaking; alcohol and sedatives slow it down. Though in certain ways essential tremor does resemble the shaking of PD, moreover, rigidity and bradykinesia are conspicuously absent, and this makes the diagnosis fairly cut-and-dried.

Striatonigral Degeneration

Still another rare ailment, striatonigral degeneration causes stiffness and rigidity, slows movement, disturbs balance, and, despite the fact that a tremor is usually absent, produces behaviors that to all intents and purposes is identical to PD.

Although this disease cannot always be adequately diagnosed

during the first examination, the diagnosis becomes clear once L-dopa or other PD medications are prescribed. In such cases, these drugs produce absolutely *no* improvement, and the person tends to degenerate no matter what medical steps are taken. Ultimately a definitive diagnosis of striatonigral degeneration can be made only by autopsy. Its cause remains unknown.

THE FIVE STAGES OF PARKINSON'S DISEASE

People diagnosed with Parkinson's disease will be anxious to know what lies in store for them in the months and years to come. Although every individual's symptom picture is a bit different, of course, and while some people remain on the same symptomatic plateau for many years whereas others decline in a relatively short period of time, attempts have nonetheless been made to categorize the stages of PD into a general rating scale. Based on probabilities and statistical data, such scales chart the chronological progress that Parkinson's disease follows as time passes and, to a degree, predict this progress as well.

Several measuring systems are in use today including the Cornell-UCLA scale, the Webster scale, and the University of British Columbia scale. Perhaps the most frequently used is the Hoehn and Yahr scale that divides Parkinson's disease into five stages and is described below.

Go over this scale with attention and concern. If the chronology rings true to your own experience, consider its implications. But remember that no one knows for sure how parkinsonism will develop in any particular human being. Jon Robert Pierce, in his book *Living with Parkinson's Disease,* says it well:

The worsening of Parkinson's disease symptoms in my own experience and with others with whom I have compared notes, does not seem to be a linear decline where there is a predictable loss of capabilities each year. Rather, it seems that the disease progresses through any number of plateau intervals, interspersed with sometimes precipitous declines which can be set off by trauma, stress or uncertainty. One would expect that once a level of competence has been lost it would be gone forever. Again, in my experience, this is not always the case.[1]

The Hoehn and Yahr Scale

Stage Zero

Medical professionals are uncertain how many months or years elapse between the time Parkinson's originates in the body and when its symptoms become apparent. Does the disease remain in potentia for many years, one wonders, "incubating" as it were? It is interesting to consider that recent medical thinking now believes that the destruction of substantia nigra cells begins in most people at a relatively young age, and that if each of us lived long enough we would *all* get Parkinson's disease. If this is the case, every living person is a ticking Parkinson's time bomb, some programmed to go off at sixty-three and some at ninety-nine.

Still, the question remains: At what point does the silent onset of Parkinson's really begin? According to the Hoehn and Yahr scale, a person is said to be at stage zero until the symptoms become visible.

Stage One

The symptoms of Parkinson's disease now manifest themselves, but on one side of the body only. A tremor may become troublesome, but only in the left hand or in the right foot. A person generally feels and acts normally.

Stage Two

Both sides of the body now become symptomatic. If shaking is a predominant complaint it appears in both hands or both legs, usually more in one limb than the other.

Rigidity now becomes more global. For instance, there may be clinical evidence of it in one arm and in the axial musculature at the same time, causing the trunk or neck to stiffen. The disease feels as if it is on the increase, and that it is, as it were, "spreading."

Despite the encroachment of symptoms at this stage, people tend to be free from more seriously incapacitating complaints such as loss of balance or immobility. After the proper medications are prescribed life goes on more or less as always.

Stage Three

Balance impairment now begins. People lose their footing for no apparent reason. They stagger and fall without provocation. Mobility problems such as festinating gait develop. Patients are unable to turn around in a small space. They incline forward when they walk or lean backward when seated. They need a small push from another person to get out of a chair. Their arms hang stiffly by their sides when they walk. They tend to forget where they put their house keys or what time they must take their medication.

In general: (1) Body movement becomes more awkward and problematic at stage three; (2) an occasional hand is needed from other people to get things done; and (3) memory and recall deficits begin to show.

Stage Four

In stage four major walking and mobility difficulties set in. Most patients cannot perform normal physical activities for themselves and require help from others. For instance, people may be unable to rise from a chair without a strong arm or a walker for assistance. They may have difficulty walking down the stairs. They may find it impossible to make ordinary sawing motions with a knife; family members will have to cut their food for them.

In general, mobility is greatly restricted at this stage, and the person requires a caregiver's assistance for some if not all daily activities.

Stage Five

Stages zero through two indicate mild parkinsonism. Stage three is moderate. Stages four and five are advanced.

While the difference between each stage is substantial, the gap between four and five is perhaps the widest. At stage five the stricken person can no longer walk, even with assistance. A wheel-chair is required. People find it almost impossible to stand up alone, to get off the sofa, to dress themselves in the morning, to undress themselves at night. Help round the clock is necessary.

The types of complaints experienced in the early days of the disease such as tremor become secondary to the more serious symptoms of rigidity and bradykinesia. Now movement seems to be at quarter-time, with every action requiring a great deal of time to accomplish if it gets accomplished at all.

Despite severely decreased mobility at this stage, patients often remain mentally alert with, at worst, some memory and recall problems. At times they will be able to perform basic physical maneuvers on their own such as dressing. Occasionally they will show sudden, unexpected bursts of energy and productivity.

Once again, realize that this rating scale is an approximate guide-line, not a prophesy. Despite its neat, numbered stages, the experi-ence of innumerable PD patients demonstrates that there are many gray areas between each stage, and that there is much room for variation, improvement, and surprise. To quote the *Parkinson's Disease Handbook:* "None of the currently used means of evaluating PD measures a patient's initiative, determination, spirit, or drive—all qualities which can transcend the patient's disability.[2]

WAITING FOR THE DIAGNOSIS

As a rule, PD is quickly diagnosed. Its signs are often clear-cut, especially when ideopathic Parkinson's disease is at work. When, for instance, neurologists are visited by patients who display an obvious lack of facial expression, who have a slight shake in one hand, blink infrequently, and walk in a bent way they often make a tentative (if silent) diagnosis within the first several minutes of the examination. Usually their assessment is correct.

On the other hand, in the early days of the ailment when symptoms are less developed, or when a person presents com-plaints that are due to several different disorders, months and even years may pass before a final determination can be made. The physician may request a second examination to ascertain more information before a conclusion can be reached. Sometimes the doctor will need added data to work with and will send the patient to a specialist or to a hospital for laboratory work. Sometimes the doctor may be stumped entirely and will ask the patient to come back in six months when the symptoms are more developed and easier to read. There are many possibilities.

If a definitive diagnosis is not made immediately, this is not necessarily grounds for worry. Many doctors are not in a hurry to begin medication anyway, even if the person clearly does have PD, and there is not the sense of urgency here that tends to accompany an acute disorder. Thus, in many instances there may be no reason for the patient to do anything at all after receiving a diagnosis of PD other than continuing to lead a normal, active life.

NOW THAT YOU HAVE YOUR DIAGNOSIS . . .

There is no getting away from it—learning that you have PD can be daunting and, for some people, paralyzing as well. What now? you ask yourself. What about my family and loved ones? How will they respond? Will I be a burden to them? And my friends? How will I adjust to this disturbing change in my life? Where do I begin?

As is often the case, the best way to start coping with a new reality is to deal with the things you can do *right now*. Ask yourself: What steps can I take to prepare for the future, both long-term and short-term? What problems will arise? If possible, avoid the "can'ts." You will think about them later. Now is the time to mobilize the "cans" and put them to constructive use. Emphasize your assets and resources. Deemphasize worry. Put fear on hold— it only restricts. Stress action, attentive coping, and positive thought. These will help you through.

Meanwhile, here are some experience-proven suggestions to get you started.

NINE STEPS YOU CAN TAKE RIGHT NOW TO HELP COPE WITH PD

The suggestions that follow are based on advice that professionals connected with the Brookdale Center frequently give to those diagnosed with chronic neurological disease. If thoughtfully followed they will help you get a handle on your new situation and assist you in laying the practical and emotional groundwork for the years ahead.

Step One: Take Time Out to Digest the News of Your Diagnosis

Now that you know you have Parkinson's disease there is nothing special you must do. You are under no obligation to run out and buy something, or change something, or see somebody. You may not even have to take medications right away.

What you *can* do at this point is allow yourself the luxury of quiet contemplation, of quality time spent alone digesting this new information, processing it, weighing it, feeling it, facing it. Discuss it with your friends, family, clergy, doctor, therapist, or anyone who helps.

It will take time before you get used to the new development in your life. This is as it should be. All changes require a period of adjustment. Eventually though, be assured, the new reality will become part of your daily existence and you will deal with it as you must. Meanwhile, make the process of acceptance easier by facing the situation squarely and by allowing this new information to filter down through your heart and mind at its own speed, in its own way, until it settles in the right places inside you.

Step Two: Remember That Your Disease Is Manageable

There is nothing to panic about. You do not have a terminal ailment, nor will your life come to a halt now that you have PD—far from it. PD people have the same life expectancy as everyone else. If you are similar to the millions of other people around the world with Parkinson's disease, chances are you still have many fruitful and productive years ahead of you. Chances are things are okay and will remain this way for years to come.

This is not to see Parkinson's through rose-colored glasses, only to reiterate the fact that the progress of the disease is indiscernible on a day-to-day level, and that for most people its symptoms can be regulated for years, sometimes even decades. Exercise routines are available that will counteract your rigidity. Medications exist that control symptoms. Special voice exercises can be used to improve speech problems. Many practical tricks exist to keep life on an even keel. PD is relatively manageable. Keep this fact in mind during moments of apprehension and doubt.

Step Three: Be Prepared for Emotional Ups and Downs

Learning that you have Parkinson's disease can be a shock. Over the months that follow you may go through a certain amount of psychological turmoil as a result of the diagnosis. You may, for instance, try to blot the whole thing out of your mind and announce that the doctors are crazy. What do they know anyway? Didn't Doctor Smith misdiagnose Jenny Jones last year, telling her she'd caught hepatitis when all she had was the flu?

Or you may find yourself getting angry at the diagnosis, and at the doctor, and the disease, and the world. It's not fair. Why me?

You may become depressed for a time and feel that the situation is hopeless. The disease, after all, is incurable, you tell yourself. Why bother? As a result, you stop wanting to socialize; or you become busy to the point of frenzy; or you feel nothing at all.

Whatever your reaction—and everyone will react differently—know that the kinds of psychological ups and downs that follow the diagnosis of any chronic neurological disease are common to everyone, and that eventually things even out. Know that you are involved in an emotional processing period, and like all such processes it has a beginning, middle, and end. So go with it, and don't be unduly alarmed if you fall victim to unusual and unpleasant emotions. Given the situation, they are normal. Try not to be hard on yourself for feeling them.

Step Four: Learn All You Can About the Disease

Most people know very little about Parkinson's disease. The daughter of one woman diagnosed with PD asked if Parkinson's disease wasn't "that sickness where your face gets yellow"? Another person read in an "authoritative" newspaper article that one out of two people suffering from Parkinson's will get Alzheimer's disease within five years.

"The first people I told I had Parkinson's disease looked at me blankly," relates Jimmy P., a PD patient for four years:

> A guy remarked that he'd heard about it on a TV special but couldn't remember what it was that was wrong with you when you got it. "That's the one they got a shot for now, isn't it?" a friend of mine asked. Another friend had heard of it, but that was about all. Another thought it was a kind of cancer—he got it mixed up with Hodgkin's disease. Someone else told me I'd better be careful cause if you have Parkinson's it's bad to go into the sun. This kind of dumb-dumb stuff got so bad I felt nobody knew anything about anything out there.

Be careful of rumors and phoney scares, of canned information and miracle cures, of superficial magazine articles and five-minute specials on TV. A little bit of learning is an *especially* dangerous thing when it concerns medical matters. Far better than falling victim to misinformation is to learn everything you can about Parkinson's disease for yourself, so that you will not be vulnerable to false claims, and so that you will be able to pick and choose your resources from a position of knowledge rather than fear.

Start now. Go to the library. Read books. Discuss the matter with doctors and nurses and physical therapists and health-care professionals. Attend lectures. Clip articles. Subscribe to magazines and newsletters. Consult medical literature. Talk to people who have PD. Talk to their families. Attend Parkinson's help groups and participate in their activities. Ask questions. Keep notes. The more you know, the more you can do.

Step Five: Seek Counsel

Seek counsel from those close to you and from those whose advice you respect. Friends and loved ones will be more important now than ever. So will professional therapists, social workers, doctors, clergy, and medical professionals.

This is not to say that you should feel obliged to ventilate your feelings with others, or that there is anything wrong with maintaining a private silence if you so choose; however, if you are the kind of person who draws strength from social exchange, heart-to-heart conversations can be valuable, both as a means of helping you put things into place and as a safety valve for letting out pent-up emotions.

Step Six: Work Closely with Your Doctor

Parkinson's medications must be carefully balanced for each patient depending on tolerance level, symptoms, and side effects. Adjustments are frequently made by physicians as the disease progresses, and this forces physicians to constantly pursue the difficult goal of minimizing side effects while maximizing symptom control.

A good relationship between physician and patient is thus a critical element in PD treatment. This relationship is, in a sense, a kind of marriage that will last for many years and that should be a happy one from the start. Ask yourself:

- Does my doctor seem well informed about PD? Does he or she seem up-to-date concerning the newest advances and medications in the field? Do I feel confident in this person's hands?

- Is my doctor concerned and involved with my condition? Do we have rapport? Do I feel rushed at his or her office? Do I have his or her full attention when we're together?
- How comfortable do I feel asking my doctor questions? Are my questions answered without haste or condescension?
- Does my doctor monitor my medications carefully? Do we have a good working relationship concerning dosages, schedules, changes in medication, side effects, emotional ups and downs?
- In times of need does my doctor see me quickly? Am I kept waiting for unreasonably long periods of time at each appointment?

Don't be shy about seeking your doctor's help. That's what doctors are for. Ask questions. Keep medical phone numbers close at hand. Feel free to contact your doctor whenever you need advice or whenever you feel that a symptom requires attention. Health-care professionals worth their salt will gladly take the time, especially in the beginning, to go over the whys and wherefores of your condition, to discuss medical options, to carefully explain all medications, and to provide support when it's really needed. If for any reason you feel that your physician does not meet these standards, or if he or she seems too preoccupied to give you what you need, find another doctor.

Step Seven: Know Your Resources

There are many resources available today that really help PD patients. Find out what they are. In the early stages of the disease your doctor will be your major support, but after a while new needs will arise. When they do, there is usually some individual or some organization out there to help.

When, for instance, certain symptoms become problematic such as slurred speech, speech therapists can be of value. If you have trouble coping with housework, homemaking agencies provide trained in-home aides. For psychological problems a bevy of professionals are available: social workers, psychologists, and counselors. If you can't figure out how your insurance works and what it covers, many insurance companies maintain a help line. Legal aid societies or community-sponsored legal groups will provide advice concerning wills and trusts (the Brookdale Center, for instance, runs the Hunter-Brookdale Institute of Law and Rights of Older Adults that specializes in helping older adults cope with legal problems). If you are having problems with ordinary household activities, such as cutting your food or keeping your balance, orthopedic equipment can be purchased from a number of different companies.

There are, as well, many organizations, both profit and not-for-profit, community and private, educational and service-oriented, voluntary and state, that specialize in helping individuals and families cope with the day-to-day problems that arise from chronic disorders. Many local hospitals run Parkinson's groups, while organizations such as the American Parkinson Disease Association and the United Parkinson Foundation offer services on many levels, both personal and informational. Outreach programs, telephone reassurance programs, companion services, emergency response systems, respite centers, medical lending libraries, and many other providers exist to help patients and caregivers cope with day-to-day problems. Find out what they are and where they are.

Outside resources really help. They can produce solutions for problems that you think are insoluble. They can answer questions. They can provide equipment and physical aids you didn't know existed. Parts II and III go into this subject in depth, explaining how and where to find the supports that will be useful for you on both a physical and psychological level.

Step Eight: Become Conversant with Your Medications

The essence of Parkinson's management is medication. Breakthroughs have taken place over the past decades that are remarkably effective and that really do make life healthier and happier for practically every patient who takes them. In the months and years to come you will become familiar with these substances. The more you know about them, the better it will be for you. They are, as it were, your life raft in a stormy sea.

Talk to your doctor. Ask him or her questions about each drug you are taking, about how it works, and why, and what side effects you can expect, about dosages and brands and the best times of day to take each medicine. Shop around for pharmacies, and when you find one that gives good service, stick with it. After a while you will establish a friendly relationship with the people who work there and they will become a solid resource for you when questions arise.

Talk to other PD patients. A huge canon of word-of-mouth, grassroots information exists around the topic of PD medications, and in many cases you will learn things from other patients that your doctor never tells you. Parkinson's groups are especially helpful. Here members spend hours comparing experiences and trading tips. The advice heard at these meetings may seem odd at times, and even unprofessional. One person at a PD group announced that when she swallows her Sinemet with orange juice it works better than when she uses water. Another tells the group that if you take Deprenyl standing up it works faster than when sitting down.

These are strange observations, and certainly nothing on the labels tells you such things. Yet when you follow these off-beat tips they sometimes seem to work. Or perhaps they don't—no harm trying. Each person's chemistry is different, and what helps John has no effect on Jane. Still, the fact remains, the more you talk to other informed patients about your medications, the more questions you ask the experts, and the more you pay attention, the better off you will be.

Step Nine: A Positive Attitude Is Half the Battle

In the future, perhaps a specific Parkinson's-related problem will bother you. Or perhaps it won't. Who knows? In the meantime, try not to worry about the future and try to enjoy your life today.

This sounds old hat, perhaps, yet so crucial is it for PD people to remain positive in the face of their condition, and so important is it that they not worry about problems until they occur, that it is worth dragging out homilies to make the point. Just remember, the emotional attitude you assume toward your ailment ultimately affects the way the ailment makes you feel. It also—just perhaps— has an effect on the progress the disease makes through the years, either retarding it or accelerating it. Many people, including an increasing number of medical professionals, are coming to hold this point of view.

In the pages that follow we will outline a wide selection of suggestions, supports, and techniques that make life for a PD person more full and comfortable. Follow these suggestions when they apply. In the meantime, bear in mind that the mental attitude you bring to your experience will infiltrate all areas of your life as a Parkinson's person, and that the more optimistic you remain in the face of difficulties, the more these difficulties will have a way of solving themselves. Whatever you do, avoid the negatives if you can, and make full use of your resources. Share with others. Don't worry about things until they happen. See your glass as half full rather than as half empty.

NOTES

1. Jon Robert Pierce, *Living with Parkinson's Disease or Don't Rush Me! I'm Coping As Fast As I Can* (Knoxville, Tennessee: Spectrum Communications, 1989), 13.
2. A. N. Lieberman, G. Gopinathan, A. Neophytides, and M. Goldstein, *Parkinson's Disease Handbook* (New York: The American Parkinson Disease Association [n.d.]), 15.

4

Medications 1: Getting to Know the Territory

Dick P. recently shared at a meeting of his Parkinson's group:

> If you gotta get one of those serious nerve diseases, it's best that you get Parkinson's disease 'cause at least they've got medications now that you can take to help the symptoms. Some of those other nerve diseases— they don't have *anything* that helps. We could even find ourselves lucky in a way. We don't have cancer or Alzheimer's disease!

Although few people will consider themselves lucky for being diagnosed with Parkinson's disease, there is a certain truth to what Dick P. is saying. Of all the many and terrible degenerative neurological diseases, Parkinson's is one of the very few for which effective and long-lasting medication has been developed. In the future, perhaps, help for ailments such as multiple sclerosis, Alzheimer's disease, amyotrophic lateral sclerosis, and the like will be discovered. Right now Parkinson's disease stands alone among these disorders as having medications that: (1) work for almost everybody; (2) are affordable and attainable; and (3) retain their effectiveness for many years.

DRUG THERAPY FOR PD

Six decades after James Parkinson lent his name to Parkinson's disease in 1817, the first useful PD medications were developed by the neurologist and hypnotist Jean-Martin Charcot. Operating from his famous Hospital of the Salpetrière in Paris, Charcot, known today as the father of clinical neurology, developed potions derived from the North American Indian shaman's herb, jimson-weed, which he hoped would give his patients relief from rigidity and tremor. On the whole, the potions tended to work. By so doing Charcot established an approach to PD medications that would be followed for almost a century. Extracting chemicals from a kindred witch's plant called belladonna (or deadly nightshade as it is known in the wizards' grimoires), scientists in the twenti-eth century were later able to synthesize anticholinergic drug agents that helped control early symptoms of PD, especially trem-or and rigidity, and these potions are still in wide use today (see Chapter 5).

The greatest advance in PD drug therapy, however, came during the mid-1960s when many significant breakthroughs were being made in the study of human neurotransmitters. Neurotrans-mitters, you will recall, are "messenger" chemicals that relay electrical nerve impulses from brain cell to brain cell and that keep the brain and nervous system in communication throughout the body.

Already in the 1930s scientists such as Otto Loewi and Sir Henry Dale had isolated a chemical which they called the "vagus stuff" (after the vagus nerve) and which they believed to be re-sponsible for the transmission of nerve impulses to the muscles of the heart. By the 1960s a number of other neurotransmitters had been discovered, dopamine being one of the most prominent.

Most important for our purposes, it was observed during this fervent period of discovery that dopamine supplies are measurably depleted in the brain of those who suffer from Parkinson's disease, especially in the substantia nigra and corpus striatum areas, and this deficit produces a consequent reduction of neural and muscu-lar functioning. It was similarly learned that an amino acid known as *L-dopa* (along with its derivative, *levodopa*) can, when ingested, be converted into dopamine to replace depleted supplies and thus return the person to near normal functioning. Today L-dopa, and its commercial derivatives, remain the most successful and effective of all Parkinson's medications.

Finally, several other medications are presently in use that help control PD symptoms to varying degrees. These include amantadine, bromocriptine, Deprenyl (in England) Eldepryl (in the United States), and various antidepressants and antihistamines, all of which will be discussed in the chapters that follow.

Drug therapy, of course, is not the only way in which PD patients can gain relief. An integrated treatment plan should include exercise, physical therapy, careful diet, vitamins, an active social life, perhaps some speech therapy and occupational therapy, a wholesome lifestyle, and a positive attitude. All of these factors, though important and at times critical to a person's well-being, are nonetheless planets that revolve around the central sun of medication.

The chapters that follow will thus profile the medications most commonly prescribed for PD. Each chapter will explain how a different medication works, when and why it works, what possible side effects it can cause, and what benefits patients can reasonably expect from its use. Before beginning these chapters, however, several points should be heeded concerning PD medications in general.

Many Doctors Will Not Prescribe Drugs for Parkinson's Disease Until a Patient's Symptoms Warrant Them

"I've got Parkinson's disease," a newly diagnosed patient thinks. "Why isn't the doctor doing something about it?" Remember that all PD medications carry a certain risk of side effects, sometimes serious side effects. And keep in mind that once a round of medications begins, it will probably be continued for a lifetime. Many doctors therefore are reluctant to start patients on medication until they find that their symptoms are unmanageable or intolerable. When this moment arrives the prescription pad comes out.

Be Prepared for Side Effects

Side effects will come, of this you can be reasonably sure. Some medications cause more than others, but almost all PD drugs produce some degree of secondary complaints. These vary in seriousness from dry mouth to mental delirium.

The good news is that in a majority of cases PD drug reactions are controllable. Perhaps all that is necessary is a decrease in dose, or a bit of juggling with the schedule, or a change in medication. As a rule, the right balance for any PD medication can be established within a relatively short period of time.

Have Realistic Expectations

Drug therapy does not make all complaints disappear; it simply brings enough relief so that patients can live an active, pain-free existence. This is a subtle distinction and one worth emphasis. Dr. J. Thomas Hutton writes:

> The goal of treating Parkinson's disease with a drug regimen is to reduce functional disability. For that reason it is important that the treating physician have an adequate knowledge of how the disease is affecting the life of each patient individually. A favorable balance is sought between improved motor performance and the side effects from medications. . . . A good general rule of treatment is to improve everyday activity, not to eradicate every sign of parkinsonism. With the exception of the first few years of levodopa treatment, it is usually impractical to mask completely the signs of the disease. Attempts to do so are fraught with increased risks of medication side effects.[1]

Wise patients thus temper their expectations with medical realities. Those with a tremor can look forward to seeing their shaking substantially reduced, but not eliminated 100 percent. Those with bradykinesia will find their freedom of movement restored, though not to the level they enjoyed before the parkinsonism began. Patients with speech problems will note much improvement; they may still, however, experience trouble being heard. Drug therapy, in other words, allows you to live your life with a dramatic reduction, but not a total absence, of discomfort.

Figuring Your Drug Costs

As with all medications, costs for drugs vary according to the state you live in, the pricing policy of a particular pharmacy, and the brand you are purchasing. The chart that follows is a general one at best, and is based on the prices of medication found in a suburb of New York City circa 1991. It will, however, give you a ballpark notion of what to expect.

These medications are expensive. A recent United Parkinson Foundation newsletter suggests that you can cut corners a bit by buying in quantity (say 200 to 500 capsules at a time) from national pharmacy chains such as Rx Allstate or Pharmail. Another way is to simply shop around. Many people think that drug prices are fixed or even that the prices are regulated by the government. Not at all. Costs for drugs vary considerably from town to town,

DRUG	COST PER 100 PILLS
Sinemet	10/100*: $72.50
	25/100: $61.25
	25/250: $76.25
Artane (2 mg)	brand name: $16.95
	generic: $8.95
Artane (5 mg)	brand name: $31.95
	generic: $9.95
Deprenyl (5 mg)	brand name: $135
Elavil (10 mg)	brand name: $22.00
	generic: $8.50
Elavil (25 mg)	brand name: $39.95
	generic: $9.95

*Fractions indicate strength of medication.

from state to state, and it behooves thrifty buyers to comparison shop before settling on one vendor.

So compare. Most pharmacies will quote you prices for 100 capsules of medication, and sometimes they will give you these figures over the phone. Whatever your approach, *do* compare and get some competitive bidding before you commit. You will be surprised to discover how large the price discrepancies can be for medications, even among drugstores located in the same neighborhood.

Why are PD drugs so expensive? Again, a recent United Parkinson Foundation Newsletter provides some interesting facts. According to the Parkinson Foundation, for instance, it takes a pharmaceutical company up to twelve years of testing before it can place a drug on the market. During this time, testing costs for safety, dosage, effectiveness, adverse reactions, long-term effects, and so forth can run up to 200 million dollars for each new drug, with some substances being tried out on as many as 3,000 paid volunteers. Once the drug is approved, the FDA (Food and Drug Administration) requires that the pharmaceutical company file periodic reports concerning any adverse side effects the medication may cause, along with a bevy of quality-control records. Finally, the FDA may require further studies by the company to evaluate the long-term effects of the drug—studies that may cost millions of dollars.[2]

What about generic drugs? They're okay if you can find them, which you often can't, though PD generics, especially the anticholinergics, seem to be showing up at pharmacies with more frequency these days. On the whole, however, generic drugs don't seem to have made many inroads for Parkinson's, one reason being that doctors feel the quality control used to manufacture generic medications is often poor, and that with an ailment as critical as Parkinson's disease no chances should be taken.

Still, generics cost approximately half as much as brand-name medications and for many people they seem to work quite well. Certainly there is no reason why patients should not be permitted to try them out. If your local pharmacies don't carry generics perhaps you can suggest that they should. Remember that a little tactful pestering often gets the ball rolling.

After a While You Will Probably Be Taking Several Different Drugs at the Same Time

Because of the many changes that occur in the brain of Parkinson's patients, several drugs, some of which complement each other, may be taken at the same time. Medication for PD is, in fact, a balancing act that the doctor is continually in the process of fine-tuning and the patient is continually getting used to. One woman tells the following story:

> After I'd had PD for several years I was starting to feel depressed every day. My doctor began giving me antidepressants to help out—Elavil— on top of my regular Sinemet and Artane. I got to thinking of myself as a pill factory. Every five minutes I was swallowing another pill. It was annoying. But worse I thought, oh my, I'm taking so many pills, I must be really sick!
>
> The doctor told me not to worry, that it's typical in parkinsonism to take a lot of medications, and that these drugs do not have bad reactions with each other, that they hardly interact at all, so it's nothing to be scared about. It didn't mean I was at death's door. I just have Parkinson's disease.

Your Doctor May Want to Change Your Medications from Time to Time

At every visit your doctor will monitor the dosage and the types of drugs you are taking. As time goes by, certain drugs may lose their effectiveness. When this occurs it becomes necessary to buttress the original medication with other substances, or even to replace it entirely.

If, therefore, you find your doctor writing new prescriptions from time to time, don't think this is being done simply to experiment. PD is a progressive disease, and it requires progressive attention and adjustment. Modifications and changes of medication go with the territory.

Pay Attention to Your Reactions to Various Drugs and Keep Your Doctor Informed of Them

This advice has already been offered, but it is of such importance that it should be mentioned again. A nurse affiliated with the Brookdale Center on Aging informed me that in her experience the most common problem that professionals find among PD patients is that patients are embarrassed about their symptoms and avoid reporting them to the doctor. According to this nurse, many patients do not want "to bother the doctor" or are afraid they will be "a pain in the neck." Thus many symptoms and side effects of medications go unreported and patients suffer needlessly.

Keep it foremost in your mind that your doctor is your most important advisor in the struggle against PD, and the medications are your greatest ally. Inform your doctor of any changes in symptoms, of any side effects, and of any unusual reactions so that he or she can modify the medications and keep you on the right track. This is a crucial point.

Know Your Medications

There are four major families of PD medications in use among practitioners today: anticholinergics, amantadine, levodopa, and bromocriptine. Each group has its own uses, its own pluses and minuses, its own side effects, and its own idiosyncrasies. The chapters that follow will profile each of these families, along with secondary medications that are prescribed for PD people from time to time. Read each of these sections carefully. Though you may not be taking the medicine in question right now, you never know what the future holds. Whatever you do, become educated concerning the ins and outs of your treatment plan and learn everything you can about the medications. A good patient is an informed patient.

NOTES

1. J. Thomas Hutton, "Diagnosis and Treatment" in *Caring for the Parkinson Patient: A Practical Guide,* Hutton and Dippel, eds. (Buffalo, New York: Prometheus Books, 1989), 15.
2. *United Parkinson Foundation Newsletter,* 1990, #2, Park I, p. 8.

5

Medications 2: Anticholinergics

THE NEUROTRANSMITTER TEETER-TOTTER

Thirty years ago the only effective weapon against Parkinson's that neurologists had in their medication satchel was the anticholinergic drug. Though joined by several bigger guns since that time, anticholinergics continue to bring symptomatic relief, and unlike some of the newer and more powerful medications, they cause few long-term problems, even after years of use. As a result, anticholinergics are often the first drug of choice for a recent diagnosis.

We now know for a fact that the human nervous system produces a large variety of neurotransmitters, and that the balance maintained between these chemical messengers is one of the primary factors that keeps our muscle and nervous systems working properly.

While dopamine is a crucial neurotransmitter, the way in which it relates to other neurotransmitters is equally important, especially to *acetylcholine*, which was the first neurotransmitter identified by scientists. Linked to our most fundamental physiological processes and especially to memory (the depletion of acetylcholine in the brain of Alzheimer's patients is believed to be responsible for the nerve tissue degeneration characteristic of this disorder), acetylcholine also acts as a sender of motor information, bearing neuroelectrical signals from the vagus nerve to the heart, bladder, and stomach. As such it is one of the body's most prevalent chemical messengers, continually partaking in an intricate electrical dance with the neurological network deep in the cellular regions of the brain. When the rhythm of this dance is disturbed trouble follows.

We now know that when a person suffers from Parkinson's disease dopamine supplies become dramatically reduced in the brain, and that this reduction creates a disharmony in dopamine's balance with other neurotransmitters, specifically acetylcholine. The result is a kind of teeter-totter effect whereby acetylcholine supplies rise abruptly and go out of their finely tuned balance with the dopamine.

Enter the anticholinergics. The word *cholinergics* refers to the chemical activity characteristic of acetylcholine and of substances that mimic acetylcholine's action. Thus, anticholinergics block the action of acetylcholine by inhibiting the process that activates it. This inhibiting action lowers the amount of acetylcholine in the brain, thus reestablishing a balance with dopamine. In turn, the restoration of a quasi-normal chemical equilibrium is produced.

THE RANGE AND LIMITATIONS OF ANTICHOLINERGICS

Of all the PD drugs anticholinergics are the least likely to produce major side effects. At the same time they are also the least effective.

This is not to say that anticholinergics are not valuable. They are, but only for certain symptoms and sometimes only at a certain stage in the disease's development. In general, anticholinergics work best during the early years, specifically for controlling tremor. In some cases, shaking in the hands or feet can be reduced up to 75 percent, and for some patients the shaking becomes so well masked that outside observers scarcely notice any movement at all.

Anticholinergics can also help rigidity, but with less predictableness and effectiveness than with a tremor. Some patients gain quick relief of stiffness in the joints and overall muscular system, but others fail to respond at all. Finally, for slowness of movement and lowered general effect (bradykinesia), the anticholinergics offer negligible relief at best. The same is true for balance problems and bladder difficulties.

Brands and Doses

While anticholinergics tend to be the first drug of choice for PD, they are just as frequently continued throughout the entire course of treatment. Dr. Herman Liprit, a physician in private practice in Staten Island, New York, says:

> Once patients get on anticholinergics, they tend to stay on them. As far as how long it is before you need another drug to go with the anticholinergics, this depends on what state you're seeing the patient in. If it's early they may need nothing else for several years. If the person is already fairly advanced when he first steps into your office it may only be months before one wants to add something with greater effectiveness to handle the rigidity and bradykinesia. Or sometimes you'll increase the dosage of an anticholinergic to its full dose before using other drugs. Usually my strategy on anticholinergics is not to go to a full dose until I absolutely have to. I usually push it up to a middle dose and let it stay there. That seems to get the maximum mileage without bringing on too many side effects.

There are two classes of anticholinergics: the piperidyl derivatives (Artane, Akineton, Kemadrin), and the tropanol derivatives (Cogentin). Although the difference between their effects tends to be small, doctors sometimes prescribe a drug from one family first and if it does not work well they try a drug from the second. Cogentin, moreover, is made up of chemicals that are more powerful than those used in other anticholinergics and is thus given in smaller dosages.

In general, the most commonly used anticholinergics are Artane and Cogentin, though many doctors prescribe Akineton and Kemadrin on a routine basis. All anticholinergic tablets are white (with the exception of Pagitane, which is orange and brown) and come in slightly different pill sizes.

- Artane comes in 2-milligram and 5-milligram white tablets with the Lederle Labs logo imprinted on them.
- Cogentin comes in white tablets of 0.5 milligram, 1 milligram, and 2 milligrams.
- Akineton pills are white, slightly larger than Cogentin and Artane, have a triangle logo imprinted on the front, and are 2 milligrams.
- Kemadrin is a small white pill that comes in 2-milligram and 5-milligram dosages with the "welcome" (2 mg) or "BW&CO" (5 mg) logo embossed on the front.

Doctors usually start patients off with small doses of anticholinergics and build up as necessary. When a drug is not well tolerated the pill can be cut into thirds and taken at several different times of day rather than all at once. Doctors will advise on these points.

Side Effects

The side effects of anticholinergics are relatively mild. Do, however, be prepared for a reduction in saliva with a resultant increase in dry mouth. This is to be expected, perhaps, as all PD medications produce dry mouth to one degree or another, with the accompanying formation of thick, sticky globs of saliva in the throat and roof of the mouth. There is a silver lining here too though: PD people who experience drooling difficulties will find these medications inhibit saliva output and put a check on drooling.

Other possible reactions from anticholinergics include constipation and blurry vision. If the patient has a history of glaucoma or other serious eye diseases, this information should be reported to the doctor *before* taking any medications. Another adverse reaction, lack of sweating, is potentially serious, especially when it leads to impaired body temperature regulation and problems with heat exhaustion. If you are taking anticholinergics and notice that your skin is uncharacteristically dry, be on the alert. If you live in a hot climate you may have to take sun sparingly and remain in an air conditioned environment. Joggers and sports lovers should be especially heedful, as strenuous activity without sweat elimination is a potential hazard. Any questions along these lines should be addressed to your physician.

Anticholinergics sometimes have a paralyzing effect on the bladder with consequent difficulty urinating, though doctors usually see this condition among older men who suffer from prostate complications. Finally, mental symptoms such as short-term memory loss tend to occur when people first start on anticholinergics. A smaller number of patients suffer mild delirium, becoming confused and sometimes reporting hallucinations. Artane in particular produces this reaction. When bizarre mental symptoms occur, regulation of dosages will get the patient back on track in a short while. If not, the medication can be switched.

PD PATIENTS TALK
ABOUT ANTICHOLINERGICS

Linda D.: I've been taking Artane along with Symmetrel for a while. It helps, the Artane. As soon as I started taking it my shaking started getting better. I also just felt better all over. Not achy. The first few years the Artane didn't cause any problems. Side effects. Then the doctor raised my dosage. I started getting a little muddled in the head. He tinkered with my prescriptions. Things got better.

Raphale P.: I got hallucinations. They came and went but never really went away completely. The doctor increased my Sinemet and took me off the Cogentin which caused it—he thought. But that didn't help. I got hallucinations from the Sinemet. Right now I take low doses of Sinemet and it's okay. No more seeing strange persons walk across the room when I'm watching TV anymore. But I have to live with my shaking increased and rigidity cause when the doctor cut down the Sinemet my symptoms increased some. I can live with it though.

Beverly P.: My doctor started me on Sinemet but I couldn't take the vomiting every day and the dizziness. So he switched me to Cogentin. That made me a little queasy at first and dizzy too, but I started to take the medication with fizz water—soda—and as soon as I started doing this the queasiness went away. I'm pretty symptom-free now after three years. The Cogentin is good so far.

Paul McC.: Artane was good. It gave me some side effects too. Very dry throat. My head was unclear and I felt unsure on my feet. Memory was blocked and short. Others in my Parkinson's group saw hallucinations and had to stop taking the medication. I myself feel that these symptoms fade after a while.

Lee H.: Cogentin worked best, but it destroyed my memory. I had to get off it. I would be feeling fine, but then I'd walk into a room and not remember what I came there for.

6

Medications 3: Amantadine

Amantadine, or Symmetrel as it is known by brand, is usually given to people recently diagnosed with PD. Like the anticholinergics, it produces relatively mild side effects; and like the anticholinergics, it is generally less effective than the more powerful Parkinson's drugs.

Interestingly enough, amantadine was first developed as an effective antiviral prophylactic agent against shingles and A_2 (Asian) flu, and it was used this way for years. Only by fortuitous circumstance did a Boston doctor named Albert Schwab notice that one of his female patients who happened to have Parkinson's disease showed dramatic improvement when treated with this substance for the flu. Amantadine was promptly commandeered by the PD population. Its effectiveness as an antiflu agent has been eclipsed, even though some doctors still think of it as an antiflu agent.

Be that as it may, Symmetrel is an impressive medication when it works for PD, which unfortunately is not all the time. It is estimated that approximately 50 percent of patients respond well to it, primarily those in the mild to moderate stages, while others run the gamut from slight response to no response at all. When it does work, Symmetrel masks bradykinesia and rigidity, and is often given as a complement to an anticholinergic, which is more effective for tremors. In combination, the two drugs can keep people symptom-free for years.

Symmetrel is not without its idiosyncrasies. In addition to helping only a portion of the PD population, it tends to work for a limited period of time only. Some people take it, say, for half a year with good results, then discover that its effectiveness has waned. After stopping the drug for a while and then using it again, they notice that the positive results have returned, and they continue through another cycle until once again the drug loses its effectiveness.

HOW DOES SYMMETREL WORK?

No one is quite sure. The most prominent theory is that Symmetrel promotes the release of dopamine from basal ganglia neurons and helps restore the proper dopamine balance in the brain. For this reason, Symmetrel is commonly classified as a *dopaminergic* drug, one that stimulates production of dopamine—in contrast to an anticholinergic drug that lowers acetylcholine production.

Perhaps so. But perhaps not too. Many scientists continue to insist that despite certain atypical chemical characteristics, Symmetrel belongs in the anticholinergic family, not in the dopaminergic. Laboratory tests designed to improve understanding of the mechanism behind Symmetrel have been inconclusive at best, and a number of theories abound. Some studies suggest that Symmetrel does not actually increase dopamine supplies per se but sensitizes the dopamine receptors in the caudate nucleus, making them more easily stimulated by small amounts of dopamine. Thus, if a dopamine receptor requires, let us say, 5 quanta before it releases its dopamine, under Symmetrel's influence the receptor will respond to 3 quanta.

It has even been suggested that Symmetrel is both an anticholinergic *and* a dopaminergic. For our purposes the important point is that amantadine works, and usually it works well. However, as with all PD medications there are side effects to consider.

Side Effects, Brand, and Dosage

Symmetrel is the variety of amantadine used almost everywhere in the United States. It is sold in a long reddish capsule, 100 milligrams in strength, and is taken orally usually two or three times a day. Often it is prescribed in combination with anticholinergics and later with Sinemet. The balance between Symmetrel and Sinemet can, in fact, be a critical one in controlling symptoms, especially if Sinemet is causing debilitating secondary reactions (see Chapter 7).

Possible side effects? There is a broad range of these, most of which, fortunately, occur in a small percent of users. On the mild side are jitteriness and/or mild depression. Dryness of mouth occurs, along with blurred vision. If glaucoma is already a problem, the physician should be informed.

Other symptoms include constipation, dizziness (especially when one stands up rapidly), urine retention, and disturbed sleep. The type of confusion and hallucinations common to anticholinergics can be produced by Symmetrel also. In fact, the similarities between the side effects of these two drug families support the theory that amantadine is an anticholinergic.

One side effect that is entirely specific to amantadine is an odd skin condition known as *livedo reticularis*. People first notice it when purplish blotches appear on their thighs or forearms, often accompanied by pedal edema—swelling of the feet. Though these markings sometimes disappear on their own, they occasionally remain after the Symmetrel has been discontinued, doing little harm but giving the legs or arms an unsightly mottled appearance. Livedo reticularis is thus more psychologically distressing than physically hurtful, inflicting no damage other than the harm it causes one's self-image, which, of course, should not be discounted. Some patients find these blotches so disturbing that they ask to be switched to different medications. Others consider them to be small payment for relief.

Janet O.: I got the spots on my legs when I took Symmetrel. They're alarming when you find them. My doctor didn't warn me in advance. I would suggest for patients taking Symmetrel that they ask their doctor about these spots. Doctors should be more conscientious about warning people of side effects like these. They can scare the liver out of you. I understand that they don't want to put ideas in people's minds. I think it would be good if they at least mentioned a few things that can happen. Not everybody gets the spots. I did though. But when they happen they can be very frightening. Then you learn to live with them. They don't itch, thank God.

Ben P.: The spots aren't so bad. Maybe I had a mild case. They are confined to my thighs which no one can see anyway except my wife who doesn't care. It's the ankle swelling that bothers me. Swelling in the foot joints and the foot. Really like they are bloated. I don't take any salt; salt makes the bloating worse. The Symmetrel is good though; it helps me feel better and gives me the feeling that I can get around more easily.

Beth A.: Symmetrel worked great for about a year. Then the symptoms came back again. I liked it cause it causes me no side effects like the Sinemet does now. I could sew and I could pick up boxes at work without trouble on the Symmetrel. I wish it lasted longer though.

7

Medications 4: L-dopa

The discovery that the amino acid, L-dopa, and its commercial form, Sinemet, can be used to control symptoms of parkinsonism represents one of the truly giant steps made in the twentieth century in the battle against chronic neurological disease. A rather common substance occurring naturally in a variety of plant foods, L-dopa is especially plentiful in the humble broad (or fava) bean that has been cultivated in Europe since the Iron Age and that was at one time even suggested as a possible cure for PD.

Though nature seems perversely unwilling to provide such easy dietary remedies for such complex diseases, during the 1960s scientific tests brought to light a huge biological secret: that Parkinson's disease results from a deficit in the brain of the neurotransmitter dopamine, and that L-dopa, a plentiful amino acid that grows in backyard gardens, can be converted by the body into dopamine and can be used to replace the quantities lost through the disease process.

Soon thereafter L-dopa arrived on the commercial drug market to thunderous coverage from the news media that, among other things, touted it as a magical remedy for impotency. For some time jokes about satyrical and nymphomaniacal Parkinson's patients chasing each other through hospital corridors did the rounds—in fact, one of the possible side effects of L-dopa can be a small increase in sexual desire—until the hype died down and it became apparent that the new drug, although not a cure-all for PD and certainly not an aphrodisiac, was helping thousands of PD people return to a normal life, even those who had been wheelchair-bound and bedridden for years.

Today L-dopa in its various drug forms is, all things considered, the most potent and successful drug in the Parkinson's materia medica. Approximately three-quarters of PD people respond to it with observable and sometimes dramatic recuperation. Improvement ratios can be as high as 90 percent.

HOW DOES L-DOPA WORK?

When L-dopa is taken into the body it is first absorbed by the digestive tract, then carried to the liver, and finally transported by the bloodstream to the brain. Here it finds its way to the dopamine-starved substantia nigra and corpus striatum cells where it is chemically transformed into dopamine. These new dopamine supplies go directly to work in the PD sufferer, regulating the mental and physiological processes that have been failing. The patient is returned to relative normalcy, at least for the period of time that the drug remains active.

QUESTION: WHY GIVE L-DOPA TO PD PATIENTS INSTEAD OF STRAIGHT DOPAMINE?

The cerebral tissue, as you know, is protected by the so-called blood-brain barrier that, in essence, is a chemical "wall" situated between the brain capillaries and the brain matter. This protective bulwark acts as a kind of neural traffic cop, allowing certain substances to enter and keeping others out.

One of the substances especially high on the blood-barrier's black list is dopamine, barred entry no matter how much of it tends to accumulate in the bloodstream or how often it knocks at the gates of the brain. L-dopa, on the other hand, is readily allowed to cross the blood-brain barrier, and once it arrives in the brain it is converted into dopamine via a special enzyme called *DOPA decarboxylase.*

Carbidopa

But DOPA decarboxylase, it turns out, is present not only in the brain but throughout much of the body. Here it tends to metabolize ingested L-dopa into dopamine *before* it reaches the brain. Being an amino acid, moreover, L-dopa easily allows itself to be absorbed into the body's amino acid pool and is quickly used up by hungry tissue in the formation of protein cells. The result is that L-dopa fails to reach the one part of the PD sufferer where it is most urgently needed—the brain.

To remedy this situation commercial drug manufacturers now mix L-dopa with a so-called *DOPA decarboxylase inhibitor* known as *carbidopa.* This substance performs the critical function of preventing the DOPA decarboxylase from breaking down the L-dopa as it moves through the body. This inhibiting action, in turn, allows the L-dopa to accumulate in the bloodstream, pass through the body unmolested, and cross the blood-brain barrier intact. Meanwhile, though it has helped "escort" the L-dopa to the brain, the carbidopa itself is not permitted to cross the blood-brain barrier and remains behind, prevented from interfering with the breakdown of the L-dopa into dopamine once the L-dopa reaches the striatum and substantia nigra.

In the early days of experimenting with L-dopa, before carbidopa was commonly used, exceedingly large amounts of L-dopa had to be prescribed for patients in order to sneak even small amounts past the decarbolyzing enzymes. Severe side effects were the result. With the development of carbidopa, however, doctors were able to reduce amounts of L-dopa from 4 to 6 grams per day to as little as .5 gram a day and still achieve the same results. Sinemet, a drug composed of an L-dopa/carbidopa mixture, is the standard L-dopa medication sold in the United States. Madopar, its European equivalent, uses *bensarizide* as a decarboxylase inhibitor; the results produced by both are more or less the same.

Use, Dose, and Benefits

Since Sinemet is such a potent medication, and since its side effects tend to increase over time, it is usually not prescribed until patients show signs of entering the moderate stage, that is, when their rigidity and slowness of movement begin to actively interfere with daily functioning. Once a person is at this stage and is on Sinemet, he or she can expect to enjoy Sinemet's beneficial results for at least two to five years without too many side effects. The length of this so-called "levodopa honeymoon" will, of course, vary from person to person. Mary De S. in Los Angeles has been using Sinemet steadily, along with Artane, for eleven years and has remained more or less on the same symptom plateau. Art G., who developed PD at the uncharacteristic age of thirty-nine, demonstrated unpleasant reactions after two years of use.

Although it helps control a variety of symptoms, Sinemet is most effective in combating slowness and rigidity. The first few weeks after treatment begins PD people are usually walking better. They move with greater agility, suffer fewer aches and pains in their limbs, and sometimes—or so it seems to them—think more clearly. Improvements in tremor can likewise be dramatic, though many patients continue to take an anticholinergic along with the L-dopa to control shaking. In some cases, however, the tremor does not improve, and on rare occasions it gets worse.

Again, exactly which symptoms improve on Sinemet is an individual matter. Some patients find that their speech difficulties are not helped at all, nor is their swallowing improved. Wendy H., a member of a Parkinson's group in New York, claims that Sinemet has made her swallowing worse, especially when she is lying down. Ron Y. notes that "I feel no change for the worse in my swallowing from Sinemet. No improvement either—but no worse. I'm still drooling a lot."

Sinemet comes in 10/100 blue tablets, 25/100 yellow tablets, and 25/250 light blue tablets. (The ratios indicate the strength of the medication.) The pills can be ground up or divided. As little as one 10/100 pill per day may be prescribed by physicians, or as much as four 25/100's per day, depending both on where the patient is developmentally on the PD scale and how well the substance is tolerated. The 25/100 pills are extremely potent and produce many side effects, and so are used only in very needful cases.

Side Effects

"If you get a lot of benefits sometimes you got to give up a lot too," is the way one member of a Parkinson's group described his philosophy of dealing with the side effects of L-dopa. In some cases reactions from Sinemet can become extremely adverse, especially after a number of years of use, and patients must work closely with their doctors to control dose and to keep a careful eye on significant change.

What are the side effects to watch for? Many people complain of feeling light-headed and dizzy in the first weeks of treatment. Others talk of a strange, unpleasant taste in the mouth, or of a sudden rush of palpitations and dropped blood pressure, the latter usually instigated by standing up too quickly (salt pills and elastic stockings to prevent blood pooling in the legs will both help here). Also, as with all PD drugs, constipation, darkening of urine, increased perspiration, and rapid blinking are common, the last symptom sometimes being a sign of Sinemet overdose.

Of all possible Sinemet reactions, perhaps the most prominent and troublesome are: (1) stomach disorders; (2) mental changes; (3) disordered movements (dyskinesia); and (4) "end of dose failure," "on/off syndrome," and freezing. Let's have a detailed look at each.

Stomach Disorders

Many people suffer nausea and vomiting from Sinemet, and they come to dread the everlasting queasy feeling it produces, even in small doses. While each person is different in degree of reactivity, the following experience-proven techniques taken from discussions with doctors and PD patients and their spouses have proved valuable:

- Avoid taking Sinemet on an empty stomach. Make sure the stomach lining is properly coated with a square meal first. This is especially true in the morning: Most reports of nausea occur at this time, usually because the medication has been taken before breakfast, or because patients breakfast so lightly that their stomachs are not adequately filled. Of all the meals of the day, breakfast should be the most hearty for PD people.

- Take medications with meals, not afterward. For many patients this practice is the fastest way of getting the drug into the system and of bypassing the centers responsible for nausea.

- Be careful of caffeine-bearing liquids, especially coffee. There is evidence that it may contribute to nausea and vomiting when mixed with Sinemet. Decaffeinated coffee or tea is a good idea, at least until becoming accustomed to the new drug. Caffeine drinks should definitely be avoided early in the day.

- When starting on Sinemet it is best to begin with small amounts and build up gradually, increasing the dose over several weeks. This approach may mean that the full range of benefits will not be forthcoming immediately. At the same time, it offers the best of both worlds, eliminating the nausea that plagues so many patients and providing a wide if not entirely complete spectrum of symptomatic relief. Once greater tolerance for the drug has developed, it can be taken full strength without stomach distress of any kind.

- Try dividing the medication into five or six smaller portions and spread these doses out evenly during the day. The lowered amounts of medication in the system at any one time will help discourage vomiting.

- Talk to the doctor about *increasing* the starting dose of Sinemet. Though this contradicts what was said above, the extra carbidopa present in large doses of Sinemet will sometimes control the vomiting mechanism in ways that smaller doses cannot.

• Some people suffer loss of appetite when first taking Sinemet. For those who are overweight this side effect can be a blessing, and is usually no cause for alarm. If patients tend to lose more than 10 percent of their body weight in the first months, however, and if appetite disappears entirely, this can be cause for concern. Appetite stimulators may help; so will the passage of time. Discuss this matter with your doctor.

• If vomiting and nausea are an ongoing problem and do not respond to changes in dosage, talk to the physician about antivomiting medications. Such drugs as Vontrol and Tigan are mild and tend to work well with most patients.

• Avoid high-protein meals when taking Sinemet. It is now fairly well established that excess protein slows down L-dopa's absorption into the bloodstream and generally inhibits its effects. It is best to avoid large amounts of protein at mealtime—meat, fish, poultry, eggs, dairy products, nuts, seeds—and to take the necessary quota between meals and/or at night (see also Chapter 13).

• Talk to the doctor about using a simple over-the-counter antihistamine to counteract stomach upset; these drugs have a natural tendency to control nausea and vomiting, and being in the anticholinergic family they help with symptom control as well. If patients are already using an anticholinergic it will probably be in their best interests to stay on the L-dopa.

• Over time the body tends to develop a tolerance to the side effects of Sinemet. After five or six months dosages that once sickened patients will produce a considerably lessened effect. Patience and time are the best healers.

PD patients talk about Sinemet and stomach disorders:

Mary D.: I find that when I take my pills standing up it helps me not get so nauseous. I don't know why; it just does.

Standing up maybe helps get the medicine to the stomach faster.

Gardner D.: Try grinding up your Sinemet to powder in a mortar and taking it with bread or sprinkled over cereal. I don't get so sick to my stomach when I take it this way.

Edna D.: I have Sinemet with orange juice or grapefruit juice or any kind of citrus juice. It's reduced nausea and dizziness and that tinny taste in my mouth since I started doing it.

Depression, Mood Swings, and Mental Changes

Some PD people complain that Sinemet depresses them or gives them that "all-day kind of blue feeling," as one patient put it. "Nothing seemed very exciting or bright when I started on this medication," says a woman patient from Los Angeles. "I felt all the time slightly on edge and out of sorts. Kind of generally blah."

Other patients, conversely, find that Sinemet increases their mental acuteness and sharpens their perceptions. "Where before I was walking through life as a zombie," says one PD person, "I feel I'm back in the human race and noticing things like I used to. The problem is that since Parkinson's comes on you so slowly you don't notice how unfocused you start to get, how . . . how shrunken your consciousness slowly becomes. I didn't. I took the Sinemet and could see the contrast right away."

The effect of Sinemet on one's mental state, in other words, varies according to individual tolerance and chemical balance. For those who become depressed or nervous from taking it the usual pattern is as follows: In the first week or two after starting medication, feelings of anxiety, restlessness, and worry develop. Mood swings are prevalent, and feelings of black dejection appear for no traceable reason at odd times of day. Sleep patterns may be disturbed, and are sometimes accompanied by vivid dreaming and nightmares. Insomnia can follow.

This condition may continue for several weeks, sometimes reaching a crisis toward the end of the first month. After five or six weeks patients' mood swings usually begin to plateau out, as their bodies learn to tolerate the medication. After several months—as a rule—the depression fades.

Other mental problems are also reported. Confusion and agitation take place in a few cases, while a tiny segment of the population experiences hallucinations and paranoid delusions. Both conditions can be remedied by a change in dosage. Delirium and even overt schizophrenic episodes are also known to occur, though these almost invariably are seen in individuals with a past history of mental illness. Anyone who has suffered a psychosis of any kind must be sure to inform his or her doctor of this fact *before* starting medication.

A few hints about dealing with Sinemet-related mental changes:

• If sleep patterns are disturbed by Sinemet, refrain from taking it in the evenings. Swallow the last dose at least four hours before going to bed.

• If patients tend to get depressed at the end of the day, as many do on Sinemet, and if patients have no plans to go out at night, a smaller dose of the drug can be taken in the evening to see if the depression lifts. Some people take all their medication during the day and enjoy a kind of mini-drug vacation at night, with a commensurate upswing of mood. Talk to the doctor about this one.

• If mental symptoms become intolerable a physician may put patients on a "drug holiday." Ordinarily administered in the hospital, patients undergoing this treatment are taken off all medications for several days so that their system can purge itself of toxic drug buildup. During this time the essential symptoms of the disease will, of course, express themselves fully and may become worse. This can be a frightening experience. However, once the doctor puts these patients back on medication the usual symptomatic relief will return, this time with the added bonus that the drug will be tolerated better than before and that its side effects will be reduced.

Drug holidays, it should be added, are prescribed not only

for Sinemet-caused mental changes but for unpleasant drug effects of any origin. Happily, a short withdrawal period seems to strengthen a drug's effectiveness and helps keep adverse reactions temporarily at bay. Drug holidays are not practiced as frequently as they were at one time, though many doctors still consider them to be of value.

• Following is some advice from PD people on drug-induced depression:

Edna: It will pass. Don't worry. You may (or may not) be depressed for a while but that's natural. You're just anxious about the new medication, whether it will work, what will happen to you. It comes and goes. You'll feel better.

Ralph: The Sinemet made me loggy for a short time. After that I felt a lot better. The cobwebs cleared.

Bette: Keep as busy as you can. I found that when I sat around moping and feeling sorry for myself about having Parkinson's and being forced to take the dumb medicine I feel depressed. When I force myself to get up and go out and visit my grandchildren, work at the library, take a bus, and things of an active nature like that I feel better. You'll have to pace yourself—though you'll find, I think, as I did, that the Sinemet gives you more energy after the first few weeks of taking it.

Dyskinesia

Dyskinesia—abnormal, uncontrolled movements of the limbs, torso, and face—is perhaps the most troubling of all side effects of Sinemet. Unlike the PD tremor with its relatively abbreviated forms of shaking, the arms and legs of dyskinesiac people move about every which way in slow, rolling, sweeping movements, as if directed by some autonomous control center outside themselves. People afflicted with this disorder twist and crook themselves into contorted postures; their arms undulate in a sometimes graceful, sometimes tortured dance. Dyskinesiac people may grimace, stick out their tongues, smack their lips, make strange faces, chew violently—each person's reaction is different.

When observers witness dyskinesia in PD patients they assume it is the result of Parkinson's disease. But this is not the case. Dyskinesia is a side effect of Sinemet or sometimes of other PD medications. It tends to occur soon after the drug is swallowed, when blood level is at its highest. Sinemet-induced dyskinesia, moreover, seems to be related to the number of years a person is on the drug. This notion is given clear support by the fact that dramatic dyskinesias are rarely observed in patients just starting on Sinemet, and that usually only those who have taken it for many years suffer extreme reactions.

Why this is so is most likely related to the fact that the dopamine receptors in the brain are somehow altered by long-term use of L-dopa and that the brain builds up a tolerance to it as the years pass. There is even some data to indicate that the early administration of Sinemet actually accelerates the development of the underlying disease process, and that premature use may ultimately be counterproductive. Many doctors thus prescribe anticholinergics or Symmetrel, first giving Sinemet only when the benefits of the other two drugs decline.

Generally speaking, dyskinesia occurs most markedly in the first few hours after the drug has been ingested. In most cases, dyskinesiac movements fluctuate during the day as a variable of dosages. Experimenting with dosage levels can help.

Some tips:

- The amount of medication taken at each swallowing should be monitored. Sometimes many small doses spread over the day are better than two or three large ones.
- The hour of day the drug is ingested may be important. Certain times may be better than others. Try it out.
- For some people swallowing the medication on an empty stomach reduces symptoms. For others the opposite is true. Try both.
- Generally speaking, dyskinesia will *always* be curtailed by reducing the Sinemet or by stopping it completely. The trouble is that once reduced the regular symptoms of PD return with a vengeance. Thus, much of the effectiveness of

Sinemet therapy depends on the doctor-patient relationship and the way in which both parties work out the balance between drug relief and drug side effects. A good working relationship with the doctor is one of the best assets a parkinsonian can have in this regard.

• A helpful strategy for working around dyskinesia is to first study your dyskinetic patterns. Ask yourself:

What times of the day are they the worst; what times are they the best?

In what ways does physical activity affect the dyskinesia?

What about exercise? Does it help?

What is the relationship of dyskinesia to eating patterns? Sleep patterns? Fatigue level? Emotional states?

What social and psychological situations make the writhing worse?

Once these factors have been studied and one has a good picture of his or her patterns, the day can be structured so that demanding activities are accomplished during the good times and the less important things are left for later.

Leslie Y.: I find that in the early morning my dyskinesia is worse. In the afternoon after lunch it improves. In the late afternoon it gives me trouble. I arrange my day so that I get most of what I have to get done between the hours of 10 in the morning till 3 P.M.

Bill P.: I had been taking Sinemet for about six years and all of a sudden I got cramping in my feet where my foot would turn, the whole foot. My ankle bone touched the floor. And dyskinesia. I went to the doctor and he said it was medication, changed it, and it's been okay ever since. He reduced the dosage of Sinemet to half a day instead of three whole ones, and put me on Parlodel. After that I had no more cramps or dyskinesia.

Finally, it should be pointed out that there is a strong emotional component to dyskinesia, and that dyskinesia becomes observably worse if patients are fearful, worried, angry, tired, or out in public for long periods of time. When patients return to the privacy of their homes, when a problem becomes resolved, or when an angry spell is overcome, they notice that the dyskinesia decreases accordingly.

"Wearing-off Failure," "On/Off Syndrome," and Freezing

A particularly treacherous side result of increased tolerance to Sinemet is so-called "wearing-off failure": A person takes a capsule at noon and by 3:30 P.M., a half hour before the next dose is due, the symptoms return in full, producing increased tremor, unsteadiness on the feet, and an overall sense of fatigue. These sensations last from several minutes to several hours, depending on when the next dose of Sinemet is to be swallowed.

A related phenomenon is the "on/off syndrome." Patients experience sudden states of immobility and weakness, often when the effect of the Sinemet is waning, but not always—a person can go "off" at any time. A patient may, for example, be talking to a friend and suddenly find her voice reduced to a whisper. She may be pushing a cart at the supermarket and the next moment find that her feet have turned to jelly—or lead. At this moment she may also "freeze"—her legs will stop working entirely and she will not be able to walk forward or backward. Or similarly, she may freeze and be unable to get out of a chair or off the landing of a staircase. Or her hands will suddenly become immobile while steering a car. There are many variations.

Sufferers of on/off syndrome never know when off times and freezing will appear, and these moments sometimes come at the most inopportune times. "I remember once when I was sitting on the toilet at a restaurant bathroom," a PD person bemusedly recalls, "and all of a sudden I just got stuck. Couldn't get up. Legs wouldn't do it for me. I tell you, I sweated and sweated for a long time wondering how I was going to get off that thing without making a fool out of myself or breaking my neck. Finally I worked my way up into a better position and was able to pull up my pants. Without calling in the calvary. But it was nip-and-tuck for a while. That was a night!"

A Few More Comments on Sinemet

Jerry K.: On-off. After the first six years it starts. After the honeymoon. Every day is different with it. Some days the medicine doesn't work at all. I've asked the doctor why and he doesn't know. You can feel fine at 10:30 and at 10:31 you start with the shakes. Tomorrow it won't happen that way.

Mary L.: I have hallucinations with Sinemet. I actually see objects in the room. Usually in the form of my mother or the dog. I'll find myself setting the table for three persons; then I'll catch myself. All you can do is say, "Oh well, that's just a hallucination" and then go on. That's all you can do if you want to keep taking the medicine.

Tina L.: I take Saltines with the Sinemet. That I think keeps me from having to vomit. I usually take my Sinemet and other medications right after breakfast. I feel that if I take it before I eat, space it out between lunch and dinner, I don't get as much stomach upset. If I take it on food I get stomach upset. Sinemet usually works in a half hour.

Bril M.: I've had Parkinson's twenty years. I started out taking straight L-dopa, the only thing available at the time. The Sinemet was much better. Tremendous. I've been taking it over a long term and it causes dyskinesia. That's the worst. The times of day it comes are related to the times I take the pill. Between two or three hours after I take it the dyskinesia gets worse. It comes on after two or three hours. It lasts about two hours when it comes. When I take the next medication it reduces. Sometimes. Up and down.

Lydia S.: I find that diet means a lot to me. I ate out at an Indian restaurant on Friday and didn't feel so good afterwards. I find that it takes a lot of efforts to digest all those condiments and spices. I have to realize that my digestion is slowed now and that I have to eat foods that are simple to process for my stomach and intestines. Plain foods mix better with my Sinemet too; if I eat plain I don't get nauseous.

Nelle P.: I take Sinemet 25/100. It gives me burning feet. Itchy. I went to a doctor and he doesn't know what it is. I was wondering if it is Parkinson's or the medication. Both the top and the bottom of the feet.

8

Medications 5:
Bromocriptine

Bromocriptine, or Parlodel as it is known in its most popular commercial form, is the newest addition to the PD drug family and is clearly a welcome one. Given mainly to patients in the moderate and advanced stages, it was originally billed as a wonder medication that would deliver the same symptomatic relief as Sinemet but would produce fewer and less severe side effects.

In actual practice, Parlodel is usually given *with* Sinemet rather than in place of it. Having a period of action that runs approximately six hours (Sinemet lasts only three or four), and not inactivated by the enzyme system the way pure dopamine is, Parlodel (and other bromocriptines such as Pergolide) acts as a cushion against the Sinemet-produced on/off syndrome, compensating for the abrupt drop in functioning when Sinemet loses its effectiveness. Parlodel also smoothes the action of Sinemet in general, especially when given in low doses. When it is prescribed with Sinemet, the Sinemet dosage can be proportionately decreased, with a consequent reduction of side effects.

As far as side effects are concerned, it is now clear that bromocriptine produces its own syndrome of reactions that can be as unpleasant as those brought on by Sinemet, especially when given alone and in large doses—but only sometimes. It depends on who is taking it and how much is prescribed. Indeed, bromocriptine is such a relatively new drug that several more years will be needed before it can be thoroughly evaluated and understood.

HOW DOES BROMOCRIPTINE WORK?

Bromocriptine is a dopamine receptor agonist. Agonist drugs in general are designed to "fool" certain cell systems into thinking they are receiving X substance when in fact they are getting Y. In the particular case of bromocriptine:

1. The X substance is dopamine.
2. The Y substance is the agonist, bromocriptine, designed to mimic the action of dopamine.
3. The cells to be fooled are the dopamine receptors in the corpus striatum to which the substantia nigra normally sends its dopamine.

While dopamine receptors are extremely selective, becoming active only when stimulated by dopamine and showing no response whatsoever to other neurotransmitters, the agonist drugs "trick" the receptors into believing that the agonist substance represents new supplies of dopamine coming from the substantia nigra, and that the receptors should now become activated as they might if a fresh supply of dopamine were being delivered. In this way the brain cells are literally manipulated into working as they would if the dopaminergic system were functioning normally.

Remember that PD begins when numbers of cells deteriorate in the substantia nigra and can no longer supply the corpus striatum with enough dopamine to keep the nervous system working properly. The difference between the action of bromocriptine and Sinemet is thus that Sinemet, once converted in the brain, actually does provide new supplies of dopamine to the striatum, whereas agonist drugs stimulate the receptors without really giving them anything new. In both cases, the end result is the same: Physical and mental functioning are improved.

Brands and Dosages

While Parlodel is the best known drug in the bromocriptine family, Pergolide is rapidly gaining favor among many physicians: Both substances work on the same principles and both produce the same good and bad effects. Pergolide, however, tends to last longer than Parlodel, requires a smaller dose to achieve the same effects, and—according to some doctors and patients—produces fewer side effects. Again, no one will be certain of any of this information until more time has passed.

For people with mild or moderate PD, 20 milligrams of Parlodel, usually in combination with Sinemet, is an average dose. Sometimes less is prescribed, rarely more, especially when the drug is given alone. Since Parlodel is a particularly strong agent with potentially significant side effects, doctors start patients on small doses and take several weeks or even months to build up to full strength. Parlodel comes in a 2.5-milligram round white tablet, and a 5-milligram orange and white oblong capsule.

Side Effects

The general side effects of Parlodel are surprisingly similar to those of Sinemet: nausea, dizziness, vomiting, dyskinesia, and low blood pressure. As with Sinemet, the body tends to accustom itself to Parlodel in a few weeks, and then the nausea becomes reduced accordingly. The dyskinesia is similar too, and is affected both by a person's emotional state and by the dosage size.

Perhaps the most alarming of bromocriptine's possible side effects are abnormal mental reactions. Dr. Jon Dorman says:

> Of all the Parkinson's drugs I deal with, bromocriptine is the one with the most frequent severe side effects, mental ones usually. More major mental disorders result from this than from any other PD drug, as far as I'm concerned. Hallucinations, semidelirium, delusions, confusion,

memory loss. This happens usually after a person has been taking the medication for a while.

According to Dr. J. Thomas Hutton, more than half the people taking bromocriptine experience some degree of confusion. This reaction is especially common among the very old and among those in the advanced stages of PD (according to Hutton, confusion is considerably less likely when Parlodel is used in the early stages or when it is taken by younger patients).[1] When severe mental reactions do take place a change of dosage will usually keep things under control. If not, the medication may have to be changed.

Many physicians give bromocriptine to patients in the later stages of PD so that they can cut back on their Sinemet and reduce the freezing and on/off syndrome that large amounts of Sinemet produce. Bromocriptine is most often given in combination with other drugs rather than alone. Dr. Dorman says:

> It's not uncommon for a Parkinson's patient to finally end up on Amantadine, an anticholinergic, Benadryl at night, Parlodel, and Sinemet, all at the same time. It's not so unusual to end up on five drugs. They each play a part, each tend to balance off each other, and all together they keep the person functioning as well as possible.

Bromocriptine, therefore, like all other PD drugs, is a powerful helper and a troubling disabler. And like the other medications, it tends to help most in the beginning and to lose its potency over time. Luckily, doctors have found that when an agonist agent does stop working another agonist from the same drug family can be substituted in its place, often with immediate improvement. This is not true for everyone, but it is for enough patients that the attempt is warranted.

Patients Comment on Bromocriptine

Nick H.: I've had Parkinson's fifteen years. I got Sinemet originally at 25/250 with four tablets a day right from the start.

Then I was put on Symmetrel and Artane and an experimental program for Pergolide. That really was a miracle. After I took it for a month or less I was a completely new man. I've reduced my Sinemet now. I used to freeze, put my hand in my pocket and couldn't take it out. With Pergolide that doesn't happen.

Susan R.: Parlodel—it seems to work fairly well except my leg starts not to work all of a sudden. Just like that. I take it with Sinemet and Eldepryl.

Tom O.: They took me off Sinemet cause the side effects were so bad and put me on Parlodel. At first the side effects were low and the helping effect high. Then some side effects started to come, especially freezing. But it's still better than that damned Sinemet.

Roz C.: Parlodel helps my Sinemet work better and last longer. I'm sure of that now after a year of taking it. I take Artane too for my tremor.

NOTE

1. J. Thomas Hutton and Raye Lynne Dippel, "Diagnosis and Treatment." In *Caring for the Parkinson Patient* (Buffalo: Prometheus Books, 1989), 27, 28.

9

Medications 6: Other Useful Drugs for PD

DEPRENYL

Anticholinergics, amantadine, L-dopa, bromocriptine—these are the big four of PD medications. Very recently, however, the FDA approved another substance for use in the United States that with some good luck will take its place as number five: Deprenyl (or Eldepryl as it is known in the United States).

In Chapter 3 we saw how the activities of illicit drug manufacturers, combined with the discoveries of medical researchers, revealed that Deprenyl produces useful antiparkinsonian effects. These stem from the fact that Deprenyl blocks the so-called monoamine oxidase B enzyme that regulates the amounts of dopamine produced in the body. By inhibiting this monoamine oxidase, dopamine supplies are allowed to accumulate more freely in the brain, with a commensurate improvement in symptoms.

How well does Deprenyl work? It's too soon to know. Dr. Walter Birkmayer, a famed neurological researcher and an early champion of the drug, believes it enhances Sinemet's effect and thus improves parkinsonian response in general. In several studies carried out in Europe and the United States using Deprenyl, however, there were few striking changes noted in patients. Some professionals even claim that the improvement experienced by users is due to the fact that the drug is a monoamine oxidase inhibitor acting as an antidepressant to mask feelings of depression, and hence creating the *illusion* of improvement.

Others disagree. Birkmayer himself, after almost a decade of research, published his clinical findings stating flatly that patients who use Deprenyl do better in the long run than those who do not. In double-blind experiments conducted at the famous DATA-TOP program, statistics support this assertion, showing that out of the 800 or so PD patients evaluated by examiners from different parts of the country, those who took Deprenyl showed greater improvement than those who used placebos. Similar experiments were done at the California Parkinson's Foundation in San Jose, showing that early use of Deprenyl can substantially delay the development of symptoms and the related need for stronger drugs such as Sinemet.

The evidence is conflicting. Some patients tell of no improvement at all; others rave of success. Still others claim that although Deprenyl has not produced dramatic symptomatic relief, it does seem to slow down the progress of the disease itself. All in all, indications are that the drug's strongest qualities are its ability to strengthen the effectiveness of other Parkinson's drugs like Sinemet and to lengthen the period of time in which these drugs continue to work. Several PD patients offer their opinions:

Claudia Z.: Eldepryl I take with Sinemet. I think it makes the Sinemet last longer, maybe a half hour longer. I think I'm taking less Sinemet because of it, and so I'm getting fewer side effects. I'm thinking that maybe I can cut down on the Sinemet.

John B.: I feel a lot better on it. That's all I know. I can't tell you exactly why. An overall kind of thing.

Liu Yuan: I find that taking Eldepryl approximately forty-five minutes before the Sinemet helps. What happens is that the

L-dopa gets to my brain much faster, and the period in which I'm "off" gets shorter. The only side effect I find from the Eldepryl is that I'm wide awake. I can go twenty hours without sleep.

John R.: I haven't found any change yet, but I've only been using it a couple of weeks. Maybe it helps the Sinemet work better. At least that's what they say.

BETA BLOCKERS

Inderal, Corgard, and other beta blockers are occasionally prescribed for symptomatic relief from a PD tremor, especially when more powerful drugs like Sinemet are not well-tolerated. While the actual degree to which tremor is reduced by these agents is not very dramatic—a person's shaking will slow slightly but will rarely be eliminated—beta blockers seem to have an emotionally stabilizing effect as well, and are sometimes prescribed for people who are anxious or whose symptoms increase dramatically in times of stress. In general, beta blockers do not play a large part in the Parkinson's medication picture.

ANTIHISTAMINES

Chemically speaking, antihistamines such as Benadryl, Disipal, and Phenoxene are part of the anticholinergics family. When properly prescribed they serve two purposes: (1) to control the symptoms of PD, especially tremor, and (2) to relax patients and improve their sleep. Benadryl especially alleviates tremor and reduces anxiety, though it makes patients drowsy as well, sometimes too drowsy to continue its use.

Most antihistamines are purchased without prescription and are among the first medications given to newly diagnosed patients. They work relatively well in the beginning and trigger few side effects. The one reaction they do almost invariably cause is drows-

iness, and patients are cautioned not to drive or perform dangerous work when under their influence. Since, moreover, they are
so familiar to most of us, antihistamines are often considered to be
nothing more than weak over-the-counter allergy medications,
and patients sometimes feel that doctors are not taking their
symptoms seriously enough when antihistamines are prescribed.
The fact is, however, that these substances happen to be effective
PD medications in their own right, sometimes surprisingly effective, and that they can be used safely throughout the term of a
person's disease, though always in combination with other,
stronger drugs.

TRANQUILIZERS

Tranquilizers, often prescribed for anxiety or sleep problems, can
interfere with the processing of dopamine in the brain cells and
actually *worsen* symptoms, occasionally producing psychotic episodes. They must be used with extreme caution, especially the
powerful ones such as Thorazine and Stelazine. Some patients
find that mild tranquilizers like Valium have a calming effect and
do tend to help lesson on/off syndrome. But at best these drugs
give temporary relief, while their potential side effects—dizziness,
lethargy, plus possible addiction—can be anxiety producers. Caution is advised, especially for long-term use.

ANTIDEPRESSANTS

The most commonly prescribed antidepressants are the tricyclic
compounds such as Tofranil, Vivactil, Endep, and especially Elavil, the recent star in the field that, mercifully, besides helping to
raise a person's spirits has certain beneficial anticholinergic effects
as well. These drugs produce sedative qualities, helping agitated
patients relax and sleep better at night.

Be informed that antidepressants do not work instantly and may take as long as a month before their full mood-elevating qualities are experienced. Tricyclic antidepressants, moreover, sometimes cause dizziness, though drugs such as Elavil tend to be more or less symptom-free for many people.

10

Surgery

Although there has been a great deal of recent publicity and controversy surrounding the question of surgery and Parkinson's disease, the fact is that this field is in its relative infancy and that the surgical option for PD remains something of a last-ditch possibility.

Interestingly, several decades ago surgery for PD was a good deal more common than it is today. The earlier methodology was considerably different from modern techniques and invariably involved some type of destruction of the neural tissue responsible for Parkinson's symptoms. One method, for example, practiced by Dr. Meyer in the 1940s, called for opening the brain and removing parts of the caudate nucleus. Over 50 percent of patients operated on did in fact improve, but more than 10 percent never woke up from the operation. Another related procedure required slicing nerve bundles in the corpus striatum, while another, the well-known *thalamotomy*, involved freezing part of the thalamus so that the tremor and rigidity might be lessened.

Although such methods were chancy and provided improvement on an erratic basis only, it is difficult to realize today what a hopeful option they offered to people faced with the choice of surgery or total immobility. Given such a decision, even the smallest postoperative improvements were counted as victories, and the glaring perils that accompanied these procedures were thought by many to be well worth the risk.

Happily, when stereotaxic surgery was developed in the early 1960s the odds in favor of surgical success improved considerably. This method involves passing an electrode into the brain via a small hole in the skull and carrying on all surgery in a small, pinpointed area, thus eliminating the need for major cutting. The technique is still in use today.

Overall, the relatively small number of patients who were treated surgically for PD through the years did fairly well. Side effects were occasionally severe, deaths did occur, but improvements could be impressive, and the future of PD surgery looked promising. Then in the 1960s and 1970s L-dopa came on the scene and it quickly became apparent that its effects were far safer and more complete than anything offered by surgery. From that time on, PD brain operations went out of style. Despite some occasional advances that burst on the Parkinson's scene now and then with the drama of fireworks (and that fizzled out as quickly), PD surgery remained more or less an orphan child of PD therapy up to the 1980s.

Then a few years ago surgical procedures made something of a comeback, mainly through the development of procedures based not on destroying nerve tissue as before but on implanting new nerve tissue directly into the brain. This approach was pioneered in the 1970s by Swedish scientists who transplanted dopamine-forming adrenal gland cells into the brain of PD sufferers. The results of these and other attempts were disappointing, even disastrous, until 1987 when Dr. Ignacio Madrazo of the La Raza Medical Center in Mexico claimed a high rate of improvement in patients' speech, balance, and tremor using his own variations of adrenal implant technique. Doctors from around the world reviewed Madrazo's data and most found his documentation incomplete and inconclusive. The mortality rate from his operations also tended to be a high, unacceptable 10 percent.

Still, a small portion of Madrazo's patients definitely did improve, even though most of the transplanted adrenal cells failed to survive the implant. Why were these patients getting better? Was it the placebo effect? Could surgeons achieve the same limited success by performing sham operations? It was even suggested that there is a kind of traumatic release of nerve growth that takes place during brain operations, and that any beneficial effects resulting from such procedures are similar to the improvement in patients receiving shock treatment. (According to sixteen medical papers written since 1983, ECT—electroconvulsive therapy—has, in fact, been used on a number of PD patients, with surprisingly good results.)[1] All of this is conjectural at best, and in general Dr. Madrazo's findings were not replicated by enough surgeons to prove his case.

Soon thereafter, Dr. Madrazo and a number of other physicians used their knowledge of surgical implant procedures to pioneer an even more effective—and controversial—technique. This method calls for removing dopamine-producing tissue from a human fetus and planting it directly into the brain of PD sufferers. Such tissue must, of course, be removed from an aborted embryo early in its growth, before the neural growth cones that join and synapse it to other nerve cells are fully matured. Not only are these young cells as yet unaffected by the aging process but once implanted they have all the built-in genetic machinery necessary to manufacture dopamine for many years to come. Fetal cells are also less likely to be rejected by the recipient's immune system than are cells taken from an adult.

The operation is performed by first aborting one or more six- to eight-week-old fetuses and removing their dopamine-producing brain cells. These cells are dissolved in a salt solution carefully balanced to simulate body fluids, then channeled directly into the patient's brain via a small tube. "We were gardening," remarks Dr. Curt Freed, professor at the University of Colorado Health Sciences Center and one of the first surgeons to successfully use the fetal method. "It's like planting seeds. When the seeds take root in the brain, we get a transplant effect."[2]

While long-term data on fetal transplants are still accumulat-

ing, reports are favorable. At a recent symposium on neural trans-
plantation held at Cambridge University in 1989 it was reported
that 31 percent of patients receiving fetal implants around the
world showed marked symptomatic improvement, while 65 percent reported minimal to moderate improvement. The more successful patients no longer needed to use Sinemet at all. There were
no complications reported from these operations, and no deaths.

However, many people remain haunted by the moral issues
that surround the implant question and that cause so much ran-
corous debate between the scientific and religious/humanistic
communities. Seven states have so far passed laws preventing fetal
cell implants. Does state government have the right to interfere
with such life-and-death medical issues? On the other hand,
should a child die so that an elderly person can live? Is abortion
murder? Where will fetal tissue be procured? How does society
put a price on such items? Will "fetus farms" soon open from
which, to use one of the more amazing euphemisms of our time,
embryos will be "harvested" on a regular basis? Certainly some
abortions occur naturally; but do such cases produce enough
"materials" to meet the rapidly expanding demand? Will a black
market in fetuses ultimately arise, complete with paid volunteers
and a commensurately higher number of abortions? Hasn't this
begun to happen in some countries already?

These and many other questions seriously trouble the waters
of the fetal implant question, with the opposing sides taking identi-
cally intractable and at times equally sanctimonious positions.
Leaving aside this thorny and perhaps irreconcilable dilemma, it
can simply be said that at the present time surgery remains a
promising but secondary option for most PD people, especially
those who are already doing well on medication. Side effects,
sometimes severe side effects, do occur from operations, and death
always looms as a possible outcome. Complications of some kind,
if not inevitable, are possible and perhaps even probable, especially among older people with advanced cases of PD who are
usually the most likely candidates for such procedures.

At the same time, not only are the results of the new surgical
procedures impressive but other remarkable techniques (such as,

among others, the implantation of nonfetal enzyme cells genetically engineered to replace dopamine supplies, or the implantation of slow-release encapsulated dopamine-producing cells directly into the brain) are being worked on throughout the world. Thus, the ultimate prognosis for Parkinson's disease surgery remains optimistic, if cautiously so, and the research goes steadily forward.

NOTES

1. See, for instance, *New York Times,* November 25, 1989, Letters to the Editor.
2. *New York Times,* May 2, 1989, C3.

PART II

Physical Activity and PD: A Practical Guide

11

Exercise Really Helps

By nature the human organism is constructed to be in a state of frequent if not constant movement. It is, as it were, a self-oiling mechanism, ingeniously constructed to lubricate its own joints by the triggering action of the stretches and pulls it moves through during the course of a day. The more vigorous these movements are, the more flexible and oxygenated one's tissue becomes.

With Parkinson's disease, however, stiffness and slowness cause patients to become fearful of physical effort; they tend to think of themselves as weak, fragile, and thus they avoid the normal rounds of exertion that active people make during the day as a matter of course. True, the disease itself causes some of these stiffness problems—but not all. Some problems are due to inactivity itself.

And what are the results? Prolonged inactivity causes sluggish secretion of lubricating fluids in the muscles and joints. This slowdown makes tissue brittle. The joints lose their integrity and the circulation slows; insufficient oxygen reaches the brain. Without daily stimulation the bones grow increasingly porous and less elastic, more breakable, while the ligaments shorten and, as it were, "dry up." A state of physical fragility and declining health results.

And yet, despite the attention that fitness has received over the past decade, and despite medical assurances that many chronic ailments can be improved by exercise, Parkinson's patients tend to underrate the value of physical exercise in general. Since they feel so weak and apathetic to begin with, their impulse is to rely on medications or on the help of a caregiver. "Why make myself more exhausted than I already am?" they ask.

The truth of the matter is quite different. A safe and well-planned exercise program *creates* energy; it does not dissipate it. In fact, *there is no other self-help activity we know of that is as helpful to PD sufferers as daily exercise, both as a means of controlling symptoms and, in many cases, of actually improving them.* Time and time again experience has proven that people who follow an exercise regimen on a daily basis achieve some form of isometric and aerobic improvement. At a minimum, they feel brighter and less lethargic after a few weeks of working out, and this, no one has to tell you, counts for a lot. Next to medication, exercise is the best therapy for PD. This chapter will help get you started.

Two different PD fitness programs are described in the pages that follow. They are by no means the only workout regimens available. In some cases, a PD exercise program will be more effective if it is designed for a patient's specific needs by a medical professional. In other instances, a particular movement may be inappropriate for those with a chronic disability such as a bad back or weak heart, and in such situations the doctor and a physical therapist will be helpful in getting the patient on the right track. The exercise programs given below can be modified at any point according to taste or personal requirement. More repetitions may be added if they help or fewer may be done. If certain exercises seem too taxing they may be skipped. Others may be added. The offerings here are only suggestions.

Note also that the two exercise programs offered below are each designed to take from twenty to twenty-five minutes, but sessions can be made shorter or longer according to need, either by editing out certain exercises or by increasing the number of repetitions. Whatever works for the individual is best.

Finally, a few important points should be kept in mind concerning exercise safety:

• Always exercise in a safe environment, in a safe way. If you are unsteady on your feet, hold onto the back of a chair while you stretch and pull. If you suffer from chronic neck problems, avoid twists or bends that put pressure on problem areas.

• Give yourself small rest stops in between exercises. Workout time is neither a competition nor an endurance contest; you are not out to set a record or to beat the clock. Pace yourself.

• Work out until you feel pleasantly stimulated, but *never* to the point of pain. After a round of exercise you should sense your blood moving in a pleasant way, your muscles should glow with an inner warmth, and you should feel invigorated and relaxed. You should *not* feel overtired, oversore, overextended. If you do, you are pushing too hard. Slow it down. As one PD patient remarked about her exercises, "Too much is no good and too little is no good—just right is just right."

• Before starting any fitness program check with your physician.

The exercises included here are designed for use by people who are fully ambulatory. A short section is provided at the end of this chapter for wheelchair-bound and bed-bound PD patients. Again, it is suggested that all exercises be done carefully, with appropriate moderation and, if possible, under the guidance of a trained medical professional.

A majority of the exercises in Set One below were suggested and described by physical therapists. To be especially noted and thanked is Physical Therapist Assistant Phil Toombs, presently working at the Newburgh Physical Therapy Center in Newburgh, New York. Phil developed many of the functional exercises listed below, and his devoted work with PD patients will long be remembered.

SET ONE: A FULL-BODY DAILY EXERCISE ROUTINE

Sitting

For most PD people the best time of day for exercise is morning. The energy is strongest then and the on/off syndrome is less likely to intrude.

Some PD patients set aside a special section of their home or apartment for exercise. Others visit a gym several times a week or exercise at a local senior center. The exercise space should be well ventilated and should have enough elbow room. Avoid cluttered areas that lend themselves to bumps and tumbles. If there are rugs on the floor anchor them firmly. A hard floor is better for exercising, but the softer surface of a carpet is friendly in case of falls. In general, it is best to avoid exercising outdoors on a lawn unless it is flat and without ruts, and then only if ample supports and hand railings are available.

Find a sturdy, comfortable chair, preferably one that is transportable and has no arms. Sit down. Place your hands on your knees. Take two or three breaths, raising both arms over your head while you inhale and dropping your arms when you exhale. Breathe with your stomach rather than your chest—stomach breathing is deeper breathing. Do several rounds of breathing in this fashion, making sure to exhale slowly and deeply each time. Then relax. You are ready to begin.

Warming Up

Let's start by getting the joints lubricated in the sitting position, then go on to the standing stretches that demand more effort. Do not, by the way, underestimate the importance of warming up before each exercise session. All knowledgeable exercisers, from professional halfbacks to Sunday golfers, loosen their muscles and joints before beginning heavy exertion. They know that to launch directly into serious pulls and stretches without first getting the juices flowing can tax the heart as well as invite strained muscles, perhaps even a charley horse, perhaps even worse. Here we go:

- Sitting in the chair, turn your head to the right side as far as it will go, then to the left. Repeat four or five times to each side, being careful to stretch only to the limits of comfortability. The neck is an area of special stiffness for PD people and it welcomes this simple, effective movement any time of day.

- Jut your chin out as far as it will go, then pull it back in as far as it will go.

- Tilt your head toward the right as far as it will comfortably go, as if you are trying to touch your ear to your shoulder. Repeat to the left side. Get a good stretch on the lateral neck muscles— but be careful, no straining. Repeat four or five times to each side.

- Make a complete rotation with your head several times in each direction. A relaxing variation on this exercise is to make your neck as limp as possible and to move your head in a slow, lazy circle, letting it drop on its own accord first to the front, then to the right side, then to the back, then to the left, and on around in another circle. Let gravity do as much of the work for you as possible. Do this exercise whenever you feel anxious and tense.

- With arms at your sides, raise your right shoulder and try to touch it to your right ear. Then drop it, relaxing fully as you do. Do this five or six times, then repeat with the other shoulder. It doesn't matter if you actually touch your ear to your shoulder— it's the stretch that counts. This exercise is especially relaxing when done with extreme slowness, taking, say, twenty seconds on each repetition. It's useful for sore shoulders and stiff necks.

- Hold the seat of your chair with your left hand and reach your right arm across your body, stretching it diagonally as far as it will comfortably go above and across the left knee. Hold for three or four seconds, then return to the starting position. Do three or four extensions, then reverse arms and perform the same movement to the other side. This movement will give you a good stretch to the intercostal muscles over the ribs and will loosen up your trunk.

- Start with your hands in your lap. Raise your arms straight out in front of you, keeping them parallel to the floor. Hold this position for three or four seconds, then return. Repeat four or five times. Next, extend your arms straight out to the sides. Hold for three or four seconds. Do five repetitions. Reach your arms straight up over your head as if making the touchdown sign and hold them there for three or four seconds. Do five repetitions. Finally, keeping your arms stiff at the wrists and elbows, reach behind you and extend your arms as far back as they will comfortably go. Hold them in this position for three or four seconds, then return your hands to your lap. Keep your back as straight as possible while doing this exercise. Repeat several times.

- Start with your hands on your shoulders. Reach up, then down to your shoulders, reach up, down to shoulders. Do a number of rapid repetitions. Do another set, this time extending your arms out to the side. Do a third, extending the arms straight out in front of you. Breathe deeply and evenly as you perform this exercise.

- Hold the bottom of your chair with both hands. Kick out to the right side several times, then to the left.

- Put your hands on your knees. Bend to the right side, hold for a moment, return to the starting position, then bend to the left. Repeat several times, making sure not to strain.

- Clap your hands rapidly ten or twenty times in a row.

- Rest for a moment.

- Clasp your hands behind your neck. Leading with the elbows, and keeping your hands on your neck, stretch your arms as far back as they will comfortably go, hold for several moments (no bouncing), then move your elbows as far forward as they will go. Repeat five or six times.

- Extend your arms straight out in front of you, keeping them parallel to the floor, and wiggle your fingers for five to ten seconds.

Then open and close your hands rapidly for several moments. Then rotate your hands at the wrists.

• Holding your arms out straight, alternately touch your fingers to your thumbs. That is, first touch the index finger to the thumb, then the middle finger, ring finger, and pinky. Now work back: pinky, ring finger, middle finger, index finger. Do several repetitions with each hand.

• Hold your hands as if you are gripping a steering wheel. Briskly turn the wheel to the left side and then to the right. Continue until comfortably tired.

• Imagine you are holding a rope with both hands. Pull it toward you to your left side for several moments, then to your right. Continue to alternate sides.

• Imagine you are gripping an oar with both hands. Row on your right side, singing *Row, row, row your boat* as you do. Then switch the imaginary oar to the left side and repeat, continuing the song. Do several times on each side.

• Still sitting, lift your right leg at the knee and extend it horizontally. Ideally your leg should be parallel to the floor, but only if it is possible to do so without strain or loss of balance. Hold this position for several seconds, then slowly bring the leg down. Do four or five times, then repeat with the left leg. Lift the right leg several inches off the floor and rotate the foot at the ankle several times in both directions. Then wiggle your toes. Do three or four repetitions. Repeat with the left leg.

• Rest for a moment. Relax. Get your breath.

• Still seated, lift your arms straight up over your head. Bend forward, stretching your arms as far out as they will comfortably reach, and keeping them as nearly parallel to the floor as possible. This movement will give you good flexion on your lower back muscles and trunk. Hold for several seconds, then return to the sitting posture. *Caution:* Do not bounce while you are extended.

Let the natural stretching motion of the position do the work for you. Repeat the same movement, this time extending your body on a comfortable diagonal to the right. Hold for a moment, then back to the left. Repeat several times, alternating directions.

• With your feet planted firmly on the floor, raise and lower your heels rapidly seven to ten times. Rest a moment, then raise and lower your toes for ten repetitions. As a variation on this exercise try lifting the right toes simultaneously with the left heel, and vice versa. Note that people with neurological disease often have difficulty making reciprocal movements such as these.

• Still seated, stretch your back and spine upward, getting a good lift on the lower torso and trunk. Keep your shoulders relaxed while performing this exercise, and extend your neck as far up as possible. Hold the position for five or six seconds, then relax. Repeat four or five times. You may wish to coordinate a deep in-breath with each upward stretch and an out-breath with each relaxation.

• Extend your right leg over and across your left foot. Hold it suspended in this position for several seconds, then return to the starting position. Repeat with the left leg. Do four or five repetitions in each direction.

• Cradle your right knee comfortably in both hands and pull your leg toward your chest. Clasp it here for several seconds until you feel a firm stretch on the thigh and back, then return to the normal sitting position. Repeat with the left leg. Do several repetitions.

Standing

Now take a few minutes to relax. Sit quietly in your chair and breathe deeply. A sip or two of water will keep you hydrated and refreshed. When you are feeling adequately rested, stand up. Your muscles are warmed up now and ready for whole-body movements.

In some of the exercises that follow you may wish to hold the back of your chair or a nearby piece of furniture for support. Some people install hand rails for this purpose.

• Take a comfortable standing position, feet under the shoulders and arms resting at the sides. Reach up as far as you can. Hold this position for several moments. Get a good stretch. Now make a fist with both hands and place them in front of your chest. Maintaining a purposeful tension in your arms, very slowly pull your elbows back as far as they will go. Imagine that you are breaking a chain or ripping apart a piece of material. If properly done, this movement will accordion-up your shoulder blades and give an excellent stretch to your arms, shoulders, and upper back. Repeat four or five times, getting good flexion each time. Some people like to take a deep breath when pulling back, and a deep exhale when coming forward.

• Holding the back of your chair or a nearby support, kick your right leg out straight in front of you. Repeat ten times, then repeat with the left leg. Next, kick the right leg to the side ten times. Repeat with the left leg. Finally, kick the right leg back ten times. Repeat with the left leg. Work purposefully at this exercise and try to avoid letting the weight of the leg determine the swing. The leg muscles should do the work, not gravity. The aim here is to strengthen the major muscle groups in the thighs, and to give a workout to the joints.

• Lift your right leg, point the toe, and rotate your foot several times in both directions. Repeat four or five times. Do the same with the left leg.

• Place your hands on your hips and do a quarter knee bend, being careful not to go down too far. If balance is a problem have a friend or caregiver keep you steady. Do four to six repetitions, or as many as feel comfortable.

• Place your hands on your thighs and slowly rotate your hips. If balance is a problem grip the front of your chair.

- Lift your left leg up high in marching position, then your right. Alternate several times. Hold the front of your chair if balance is a problem.

- Bend over at the hips and comfortably let your arms dangle in front of you. Without bouncing, reach down and comfortably try to touch your toes. Then stand up again. It is not necessary to actually touch your toes, just to get a good stretch in the back of your legs. You may even find it is easier to bend your knees while you do this exercise so that your back is not strained. This movement is especially beneficial for increasing mobility of the spine and hips—two areas that tend to stiffen up for PD people—and for achieving good flexibility in the trunk area.

- In the standing position, with your legs planted firmly on the floor, twist slowly from one side to the other, swinging your arms while you turn. Don't force this one; if you have any doubts concerning your back or hips, avoid it. This exercise is helpful in maintaining the mobility of the trunk and hips.

- Stand in front of your chair. Sit down, then quickly stand up again, sit down again, stand up. Repeat several times if possible.

- Now simply walk in place for two or three minutes, briskly swinging your arms at your sides and breathing deeply.

Cooling Down

Sit down. Rest for a moment. The major part of the workout is now over. You may be a bit winded so take several moments to breathe deeply and relax. When you feel adequately rested begin the cooling-down exercises.

These, briefly, include a selection of the seated exercises plus several new ones:

- Turn your head from side to side.
- Move your head to your shoulder.
- Rotate your head in both directions.
- Hunch and drop your shoulders.

- Reach and stretch your arms diagonally across your body.
- Lift your arms up, to the side, and to the front.
- Put your hands up and touch your shoulders, doing rapid repetitions.
- Pull your knee to your chest.
- Bend forward in your chair.

Finish with a set of facial calisthenics, valuable for combating "Parkinson's mask" and for keeping elasticity in the muscles of the eyes, nose, forehead, and mouth:

- Open your mouth as wide as possible, say "Ahhhhhhh," and hold for four or five seconds. Close. Repeat several times.

- Scrunch up your face, wrinkling your forehead, eyes, nose, and mouth. Hold for four or five seconds, then release. Repeat several times.

- Wiggle your nose for several moments, then wrinkle it. Repeat several times.

- Wiggle the muscles in your ears for several moments.

- Stick your tongue out as far as it will go and hold for several moments. Repeat several times. Stick it out the right side of your mouth, hold, then the left. Try to touch your nose with your tongue.

- Pucker up your mouth and whistle a tune.

- Close your eyes tightly, hold, then open wide. Alternate several times.

- Massage your entire face: the scalp, forehead, nose, all around your ears and temples. Massage over the eyes, the lips, chin, and cheekbones.

- Smile broadly and say "Eeeeeeee." Hold for several moments, then frown broadly. Alternate several times.

- Raise your eyebrows up and down (Groucho Marx style) eight to ten times. Do several sets.

• Holding your head still, move your eyes as far to the right as you can, hold for a moment, then to the left. Then up and down. Repeat several times.

• Roll your eyes round in your head. Try to get as wide a circle as you can in both directions. Repeat several times.

• Click your teeth together approximately fifty times.

• Now take several deep breaths, sit quietly, and relax for several minutes.

SET TWO: ADL EXERCISE PROGRAM FOR DAILY LIVING

The following exercises, many of them worked out by members of the Nyack Hospital Parkinson's group, are designed to imitate the natural movements that people make during the course of an active day: putting on a shirt, raking leaves, washing hands. They are known as ADL exercises—activities of daily living.

All of us at one time or another, for example, are forced to negotiate a set of steps. There is thus an ADL exercise here that calls for marching in place, with high strides and swinging arms. The purpose of this movement is to put the joints through their full range of motion, to strengthen the muscle groups used in everyday activities, and at the same time to improve stair-climbing skills. All the other ADL exercises featured here perform a similar double function.

The following ADL exercises can be done in place of Set One or, if you wish, as a complement to it. Many people alternate, doing Set One one day, Set Two the next. Like all exercise programs it is strongly advised that you warm up first before beginning. Start with the sitting warm-ups presented in Set One above, and then move on to the following exercises:

ADL Dressing Exercises

• Sit in a chair with your hands hanging loosely at your sides. Lift your arms straight out in front of you, then reach down and touch your toes. Repeat eight to ten times. This exercise simulates putting on a pair of shoes.

• Sit in a chair. Reach down, grip your ankles, and slowly run your hands up from the ankles to your knees (or higher if you wish), then back down again. Repeat eight to ten times. This exercise simulates pulling on a pair of socks.

• Stand straight with hands at your sides. Place the back of your hands on the back of your thighs. Slowly slide your hands up your legs to your waist and then down again. Repeat eight to ten times. This movement simulates pulling up a pair of pants.

• A variation on the last exercise: Procure a wooden pole approximately 3 feet long and 1.5 inches thick. Any lumber yard or orthopedic supply store will have one. Standing straight, hold the pole against your buttocks and roll it up and down the small of your back. This movement will be similar to the one above, though the rolling action will give you more stretch.

• Stand straight. Hold your hands over your head for several moments, then slowly bring them down the sides of your body until they rest at your sides. Repeat eight or ten times. This exercise simulates pulling on a shirt.

• An exercise especially for women: In a standing position, hold your hands in front of your chest. Now slowly pull both elbows back as far as they will comfortably go. Get a good stretch on the arms and shoulders as you do, then slowly bring your hands back to your chest. Repeat several times. This movement simulates putting on a bra.

ADL Bathroom Exercises

• Sit. Grip the sides of the chair with both hands. Using your arms as well as your legs, slowly push yourself up to a standing position. Repeat several times. This exercise simulates getting off a toilet.

• Stand. Crook your arms in front of you and bend over at the waist. Remain in this position for several moments, then straighten up. Repeat several times. This movement simulates bending over a sink.

• Stand. Rub your hands briskly together for several moments. This movement simulates soaping your hands.

• Stand or sit. Hold your arms extended in front of you with palms parallel to the floor. Simultaneously (or one at a time if you prefer) rotate your hands at the wrists half a turn, first to the right, then to the left. This movement simulates turning on a water faucet.

• Stand straight. Place both hands on top of your head. Slowly run your hands down the back of your neck and then up to the top of the head again. Repeat eight to ten times. This exercise simulates brushing or combing your hair, a movement that is difficult for many PD people.

General Ambulation, Reach, and Dexterity ADL Exercises

• March in place. Lift your feet high and swing your arms. Continue for several minutes, or for as long as you feel comfortable performing this action. Marching in place simulates the act of walking up and down stairs.

• In a standing position raise both hands over your head and stand on your tiptoes. Hold for several moments, getting a good stretch on your arms, legs, and calves. Repeat several times. If balance is a problem have someone help you. This exercise simulates reaching for an object on a shelf.

• Hold your arms out straight, parallel to the floor. Wiggle your fingers for several moments, open and close your fists, then touch the fingers to the thumb in rapid alternation. These movements simulate many common hand actions such as gripping an object, turning a page, or holding a pen.

- Assume a fencer's position, with one leg forward and one back, one arm extended straight out as if pointing a sword at your opponent, one at your side. Making sure your legs are planted far enough apart to provide a firm base, gently lunge forward as if thrusting with the sword, then back again. You should feel a comfortable stretch on your calves and thighs as you make this movement. Repeat as many times as you like. This exercise simulates many general movements made during the day such as using a vacuum cleaner, opening a door, or pushing against a heavy object.

- Stand. Hold a curtain rod or wooden dowel as if it were a broom and make sweeping motions with it. This movement simulates sweeping a floor.

Do It Yourself

The beauty of ADL exercise is that you can tailor-make them to suit your personal needs.

Martha G. is a waitress with Parkinson's disease. She spends much of the day standing behind a counter, and so she has worked out ADL exercises that strengthen her calves and hips. June C. has trouble getting in and out of a car. During her exercise session she concentrates on sitting in a chair and pivoting from side to side, as she might if she were climbing out of a front seat. Both worked these exercises out according to their needs. You can do the same.

Other Exercises

Besides the formal exercise programs presented above, there are a number of other wholesome and accessible physical activities that will gain you more or less the same ends. These include:

Walking

Of all natural exercise walking is no doubt the most popular and useful. Besides oxygenating the whole body it gets many muscle groups working at the same time and stimulates the cardiovascular system, yet does not put undue stress on the joints or skeletal system as does jogging.

Take a good walk at least once a day and preferably twice. When shopping bring a marketing cart with you to the store and walk home. After dinner get into the habit of taking a short stroll. Some PD patients like to take their exercise in malls or parks early in the morning when the walkways are clear and there is no danger of bumping into other people. Bring along a friend to encourage you to take big steps.

Walking is underrated as an exercise for Parkinson's disease, and this is a shame. All professionals agree it is one of the best ways for elderly people to stay in shape.

Swimming

Water suspends exercisers in a gravity-free medium, giving them increased mobility and providing a natural source of resistance that allows gentle but vigorous exertion for every part of the body. Swimming puts the joints through their full range of motion and offers a stimulating workout for the cardiovascular system. Water, moreover, is a healing substance in its own right—cool, refreshing, therapeutic. Even a five-minute dip can lift your spirits.

Swimming laps is, of course, ideal, though benefit can be derived simply from doing a few underwater knee bends and squats, by kicking gently while holding the side of the pool, or by treading water. Movement-impaired PD patients can get their swim time by wearing small inflatable "floaties" that slip onto the arms and keep swimmers buoyant without need for paddling or life jackets. Floaties can be purchased at any variety shop or children's toy store.

Exercise Equipment

Exercise equipment can be extremely useful for PD people, especially in the early stages. Automatic cyclers, rowing machines, walking and jogging equipment all help. Simply procuring a soccer ball or inflatable ball and tossing it around every day also helps. Incorporate five or ten minutes of such activity into your daily workout if possible.

For people with restricted mobility, small portable cycling machines can be purchased that take a good deal less effort to peddle than larger models and that can be used with the hands as well as the feet. This and similar pieces of equipment can be purchased from several orthopedic supply stores including Cleo (3957 Mayfield Road, Cleveland, Ohio, 44121, toll-free 800-321-0595).

Exercises for the Wheelchair-Bound and Bed-Bound

Since people confined to wheelchairs are prone to physical problems caused by chronic inactivity, it is especially important that they be kept on a regular exercise regimen. Many of the simple sitting exercises featured above can be used by the wheelchair-bound as well. Patients must be careful not to strain, but at the same time be sure that they get at least 15 to 20 minutes of physical stimulation daily.

Bed-bound patients offer a more serious challenge, with contractures leading the list of probable difficulties. Contractures are caused by shortening of the ligaments and tendons that, in turn, result from inactivity. These cramping spasms are extremely painful and sometimes force patients to assume fetal positions. The following stretches can be administered to the bed-bound by caregivers. They will put most of the patient's major joints through their full range of motion:

- Lift the patient's right leg as far up from the bed as it will go. Hold it for several seconds, then slowly bring it down. Repeat for the left leg.

• Lift the patient's right leg and rotate it at the ankle several times. Repeat with the left leg.

• Lift the patient's right leg, bend it at the knee, and push it in flush to the chest. Hold for several moments, then straighten the leg. Repeat with the left leg.

• Lift the patient's right leg and cross it over his or her body, giving the leg a good diagonal stretch as you do. Hold this position for several moments, then return. Do the same with the left leg.

• Stretch the patient's right arm over his or her head. Rotate the arm in its socket in both directions, then at the wrist. Continue until this movement becomes slightly uncomfortable for the patient. Repeat with the left arm.

• Lift the patient's head off the pillow. Gently pull it upward away from the shoulders, hold, release. With the patient's head on the pillow, turn it to the right, then to the left. Repeat several times.

• Encourage the patient to take ten deep breaths. Repeat several times each day.

Some Final Tips

Here are some final tips to maximize exercise time:

• Exercisers find that background music helps their sense of rhythm and makes the time pass more quickly. Favorite background music includes waltzes, marches, polkas, jazz, and easy listening.

• Drink plenty of water while you exercise. It will make your muscles work at top form and will keep you well hydrated.

• Pay attention to extremes of temperature. If the weather is especially hot, exercise in an air-conditioned room. If it is very cold, stay indoors.

- Wear loose-fitting clothing when you exercise. Sweat togs or baggy shirt and pants are fine. Be careful of loose cuffs; they easily get caught underfoot.

- If you're attempting to strengthen an arm or leg, cuff weights will help. Speak to your doctor or a physical therapist about this one first.

- For the caregiver: PD people with balance or vision problems may need supervision. Stay close while they exercise. Be prepared to catch them if they become disoriented. Don't be shy about suggesting caution or telling the person to hold the back of a chair for support.

- Let the daily activities of life become exercises as well. When pulling a sweater or shirt over your head hold your arms up for several extra beats and give them a good stretch. Make bending down to tie your shoes into a toe-touching session. When watching TV, rotate your hands and wiggle your fingers. When lying in bed, perform leg lifts. When reaching for an object on a shelf, give extra extension and flexion to your shoulders, arms, and back. When sweeping, mopping, folding, or raking, become aware of the muscle sets involved and provide them with a good stretch. Every little bit helps.

PART III

Everyday Hints for Living with Parkinson's Disease

12

Managing 1: Tricks, Techniques, Hints, and Common-Sense Coping Maneuvers to Help Deal with the Daily Problems of PD

As any person suffering from Parkinson's will tell you, it is the daily ups and downs that mark the heart of the struggle. "Parkinson's is always with you," one patient remarks. "Unpredictable. Persistent. The only pattern you can be sure of is its constancy. You know each morning when you wake up that the shaking and stiffness will be there, just like the sun and the trees outside your window. They're going to be there bringing new trouble of some kind—of that you can be sure."

Day to day there are the inevitable tremors, the sudden off times, the fear of falling, the struggles of sorting, cutting, and swallowing what seems like a hundred pills a day. Life with Parkinson's disease is not a barrel of laughs. At the same time, life with Parkinson's disease goes on. Patients manage; things more or less get done in a more-or-less normal way. With or without handicaps, one must still deal with buying groceries, paying the bills, caring for grandchildren, preparing dinner, making do. And the good news is that although the symptoms of PD cannot be eradicated, there are many tricks, shortcuts, and common-sense coping maneuvers about which your doctor may or may not have told you. They are known mostly to those at the center of things: the parkinsonian patients themselves. As the proverb says, "Ask the patient, not the doctor."

The information in this part of the book is thus gathered from talks and interviews with PD people, many of whom have overcome enormous challenges, and a majority of whom, thanks to their ingenuity and persistence, have succeeded in organizing the details of their lives in a manageable way. Complementing this information is an offering of hands-on experience gathered from the caregivers of PD people, along with counsel from physicians, nurses, physical therapists, social workers, and occupational therapists who are connected with the Brookdale Center or with other medical institutions.

Read the chapters in Part III carefully. If the advice speaks to your needs, try it on for size. It is culled from a large pool of both professional and grassroots knowledge. It has helped thousands of other people who are in the same boat as yourself. If, on the other hand, it does not apply, leave it and go on to parts of the chapter that are more useful. Somewhere in this section you will find a shoe that fits.

Most important, remember that no matter how baffling or overwhelming an obstacle may seem, nine times out of ten a method for managing it does exist. The method may not be perfect. It probably won't solve the problem entirely, but it will help. And in this ball game a little help is a lot.

GAIT PROBLEMS

When starting to walk, the first few steps are the hardest for PD people. Sometimes the feet freeze or the ankles go stiff, and the only way the legs seem to work is by taking shuffling little steps that become progressively smaller and faster as they go—festinating gait—and that cause the person to walk frantically in place or to tumble forward. Sometimes the feet won't move at all. Or, conversely, they can't be stopped once they are in motion, and uncontrolled momentum sends one sprawling.

Walking has been described as the process of "controlled forward falling," and indeed, if you watch non-Parkinson's people you will see that their bodies incline slightly forward as they walk and that they shift their weight slightly from side to side in an almost metronome-like rhythm, as if to constantly correct their balance with each step.

PD people do not make these subtle sideward shifts and forward inclinations. Their walking is controlled by their legs alone without the normal fluidity of motion in the upper torso, chest, shoulders, arms, and head. If you draw an axial line through the center of a PD person's body you will find that the spine remains almost entirely perpendicular while walking, and that swaying is minimal. This lack of rhythm and compensatory check against gravity results from rigidity coupled with the bradykinetic difficulty of initiating movement. The upshot is that it imperils a person's balance and makes gait disorders one of the major impediments facing PD patients. To begin, it is necessary to master certain fundamental compensatory walking skills.

Five Basic Rules for Better Walking

1. When you are about to take your first step from a standing position, make sure your feet are at least 8 to 10 inches apart and that they are planted firmly on the ground. Never take an initial step forward when your feet are close together.

2. Push off with as much momentum as you can muster on the first step. Concentrate. Reach. If you get a good first step the rest will be good too.

3. When you take your initial steps, place your heel on the floor first, then your toe. Always follow this order. Never toe-heel, as some parkinsonians do. It may even be necessary to exaggerate these steps into slow, dramatic movements: heel, toe, heel, toe, heel, toe! Don't feel self-conscious about it. After a while it becomes automatic.

4. Don't lean too far forward. The tendency for PD people to walk with their weight distributed ahead of their stride leads to shuffling and forward propulsion. Keep your center of gravity over your pelvic region, and be on guard against stooping.

5. Consciously command yourself to take long, steady strides. Let your mind be the boss. Move yourself first, as it were, with your thoughts, *then* with your muscles.

"Will" Your Movements with Your Mind

Because the central "feedback loop" connecting the brain and body is disturbed by dopamine reduction, patients often feel disassociated from their bodies, as if their bodies belonged to someone else. "Sometimes I lift my hand up," remarks Libby F., a Parkinson's patient for eleven years. "When I do I mentally refer to it as *the* hand, not *my* hand. It feels like it is someone else's hand, not my own."

Because of this strange body-mind separation it becomes necessary for PD people to literally "will" their movements rather than to rely on their automatic reflexes to do it for them. This willing originates in the conscious mind and, as Libby F. explains, is communicated to the body via direct mental command:

> I tell my hand, *the* hand, to move. I have to give my body commands.
> I have to order. I have to think about each and every move I make. How
> do I get my feet moving? I ask myself. Well, I answer: First I arrange
> *the* feet under me and spread them wide to give myself a firm base. Then
> I relax *the* feet. Then I tell *the* feet to take a step. Then another, and
> another. I tell *the* feet to really stride out, not to take little steps. There.
> Job done. I'm walking okay. It takes a while doing it this way but my
> hands and feet *will* listen. I just have to remember to give them the
> orders in the first place—that's what's most important.

Don't Talk While You Walk

PD people have difficulty performing more than one physical action at a time. They may have trouble, for instance, opening a door with one hand and putting on a hat with the other. Patients should thus maximize their energy and concentration by not talking when they are walking, especially when taking the first few steps. Instead concentration should be placed on balance and on the feet. Talk only when seated or when forward momentum has been gained.

Break Up the Distance into Segments

If you are walking from the bedroom to the kitchen and must pass through several rooms to get there, don't hesitate to take short rest stops along the way. You can even plan your movements from room to room ahead of time, factoring in these small relaxation periods.

Begin by standing up, getting the proper forward momentum, and walking to the door. At the doorway pause a moment and hold the knob. Continue on to the next room, pushing off against the doorway for momentum and being aware of where the support objects are like tables and chairs in case you need them. At the next door pause again, then continue to your destination. Slower is better for a PD person. Consider this statement an axiom.

Slower Is Better

"I'd like to see persons with PD turn up the awareness level when they walk, and become more aware of their movements," says Phil Toombs, physical therapist. He continues:

> At the same time, to slow it down too. Slow is safe. Take nice slow steps as opposed to fast shuffling. Get heel-toeing, and pick up the feet better. If patients become conscious of what they're doing and if they do it carefully, systematically, with a purpose, they definitely can improve their gait. The shuffle approach takes the least amount of muscle activity, so the patient is going to gravitate towards doing it that way. But

that's a short cut. It's better to slow it down a bit and to extend each step, to tell yourself to take nice healthy forward strides, to do all this consciously—intentionally. We are all set in our ways—but increasing our awareness will help.

More Tips for Gait Improvement

• Keep your shoulders square when you walk. Do not let one shoulder droop at the expense of the other.

• Rock back and forth several times to build up momentum before attempting to step forward.

• Think "center" when you walk. Place your attention in the middle of your body, specifically in your navel area. Keep your concentration fixed here and imagine that you are in the absolute inner balance point of yourself. This is a trick from the oriental martial arts.

• Make use of cadence counts when trying to establish forward momentum—"one, *two;* one, *two;* one, *two!*" For reasons not entirely understood, counting out loud builds rhythm and momentum. The military practice of beating a drum or marching to accented tunes—"You *had* a good home and you *left,* your *right!*"—is a helpful model to consider.

• High sneakers are thought by some PD people to be the best shoes for walking. Their rubber soles generate excellent traction on slick surfaces, they are comfortable, and the raised padding at the heels supports the heels and ankles. If lacing sneakers is a problem, varieties are made that snap shut with Velcro. (Using Velcro instead of laces or fasteners is, in general, a good policy.) Other people find it easier to walk in shoes with leather soles. Leather is an excellent material on resistant floor surfaces like rugs and mats, though smoother surfaces such as polished wood or shiny tile may cause slippage problems. Experiment and see which is best for your needs. If you prefer leather, bowling shoes are the best bet. They offer the easy slide of leather and the traction of rubber.

• To help people overcome a tendency toward forward propulsion, certain types of orthopedic shoes feature specially designed soles and lowered heels. Ask your doctor, physical therapist, or occupational therapist where to purchase them.

• If you are having difficulty initiating your first few steps you may be trying too hard. Instead of redoubling your efforts, relax and think of any pleasant subject that does not have to do with walking. Entertain yourself this way for several minutes, then return to the task. You may find the going is easier now.

MAINTAINING BALANCE, PREVENTING FALLS

"I was standing by the bathroom sink reaching for some Visine," says a PD woman. "The next thing I knew I was on my rear end. I just fell—went plot! No warning. Nothing pushed me. Just fell."

Spills and tumbles are serious business for brittle-boned elderly people. When they occur they can initiate a cycle of injury and reinjury that may ultimately be played out in the hospital ward or even on the operating table. Although only 6 percent of falls actually result in fractures among seniors, 75 percent of the home accidents that lead to hospitalization in the United States take place among the over-sixty-five population. That's serious business. How can one avoid falling?

The Paradox of PD

To begin, realize this surprising paradox: Statistically speaking, parkinsonians are at the highest risk of injury when they are ensconced in the security of their own homes. They are at the least risk when out in the world meeting other people, visiting, browsing, participating. Just as a tremor improves when a person's limb is in motion and worsens when it comes to a rest, so this becomes a metaphor for the PD patient's plight: Activity improves the condition; lack of activity makes it worse.

What strange cross-purposes are served by a disease that at

once improves with activity and yet does its best to discourage activity in its sufferers? The answer is not known, of course, though it is theorized that the areas of the brain affected are also the parts responsible for our most habitual muscular actions, so that whatever sedentary tendencies we may already have are exaggerated by the disease.

Be that as it may, a critical step PD people can take to prevent balance loss is to remain physically active and socially involved. This may sound like a contradiction, as extra activity should theoretically increase a person's chances of falling. In actual fact, it appears not to. It appears to improve the balance faculty, not worsen it. One must be careful, of course. Yet activity does seem to help. "Vegetating at home is a sure invitation to an accident," remarks one PD person. "Withdrawing guarantees that you'll decay," remarks another.

Be Aware of the Things That Can Make You Fall

These will differ from person to person, though there are hazards that cause trouble for everyone. These include:

- Loose rugs, slippery surfaces, all general round-the-house hazards
- Fatigue; letting oneself become too tired
- Trying to turn or pivot too quickly
- Impaired vision
- Taking medication too soon or too late
- Overdosing or underdosing on medication
- Standing with one's legs too close together
- Being in too much of a hurry
- Doing more than one thing at a time

Let's have a look at all of the above.

Make Your Home Fall-Proof

Prevention is the best cure. Look around your house. There are probably many things you can do to create "cushions" for yourself or for the patient should a fall occur. Part of Chapter 14 is devoted to the many things that can be done in this regard.

Taking Rests Will Help You Keep Your Balance

Loss of balance is a variable of fatigue: The more tired one becomes, the more likely one is to fall. To work against fatigue-induced falls take regularly timed breathers in the midst of activities. If you are at a workbench, or planting a garden, or filing papers, stop for a moment, sit down, take a few deep breaths, unwind, rest, and then continue.

Don't be shy about it either. If you are working with other people explain to them that you have Parkinson's disease and that you must not push too hard. They will understand. Whatever the case, keep reminding yourself to take frequent breaks. This little trick has worked wonders for many people.

Vision Problems

Falls are often caused by poor vision. A person reaches for a book on a shelf, misjudges the distance, and tumbles. Remember, the PD person's sense of balance is a good deal more delicate than the nonparkinsonian's, and the slightest outside force throws it off. Couple this fact with the following realities about PD and vision:

1. In some cases, the ocular muscles lose their fluidity, causing a PD person's eyes to move in irregular shifts.
2. Lack of blinking irritates the eyes and causes blurring.
3. The ability to see at night diminishes.
4. Some PD patients complain of difficulties adjusting their cycs to changing light levels, of problems with spacial judgment, and of an overall reduction in the field of vision.

Put all these factors together and you have a situation rife with possibilities for equilibrium loss. You must ask yourself: Has my vision gotten worse lately? Do I have trouble seeing at nights? Do my eyes hurt more than usual? Am I seeing double or blurred? Do I need glasses? Do I need new glasses? Are there certain situations in which I should move more slowly, trusting my eyes less and my experience more? In what ways can I protect myself against errors of faulty vision?

Watch Your Medications

Several PD medications make patients feel dizzy and/or produce dyskinesia. Both these side effects increase the likelihood of falls. If you have been falling frequently, chances are something is amiss with your medication. Perhaps the dosage is too strong, or too weak. Consult with your physician. The solution may be as simple as altering the dosage.

How to Turn Around

Many falls occur when people attempt to turn around, or to make a sudden change of direction. Be especially careful when any type of pivotal movement is called for. The following routine describes the proper turning technique:

1. Plant your feet directly beneath your shoulders before you begin your turn.

2. Lift one foot and place it several inches behind you, turning your body slightly in the direction of the turn and leading with your head. As you turn, imagine yourself to be moving round a pole or central axis.

3. Pivot on your back foot and bring the other foot a few inches around with a single small step.

4. Take a second step back with the pivot foot, then move the other foot around another short distance. Repeat this sequence, taking seven or eight small steps to complete the turn.

5. Don't hurry. Be aware that you are especially vulnerable to falls at this moment. Make sure your whole body turns as a unit. Give turning the caution and attention it deserves.

"I take at least eight steps when I turn," says Libby Fine, a group leader, exercise therapist, and participating PD member of the Englewood, New Jersey, Parkinson's group:

> I am consciously careful. Heels down first, then pivot, turn carefully. Small step, small step, small step around, and easy does it. If I feel myself shaky while I'm turning I give a little and sway with the movement. I try to remain flexible, to go with the swaying. I don't fight it. I also make sure that there is an object nearby to hold onto when I'm turning in case I should freeze or feel the sudden need for something solid to grab.

Keep Your Base of Support Wide at All Times

PD patients tend to keep their feet close together when they stand, to incline backward (or sometimes forward), and to lean to one side. All three habits invite falls.

To overcome these postural tendencies, keep a wide stance with your feet separated a distance of from 8 to 12 inches and your knees slightly bent (not locked). If you are about to perform an action that requires strength and exertion, widen your stance even more. Or, if the situation warrants, try putting one leg behind you and one leg in front to brace yourself. Experiment. See what posture provides the best feeling of balance and then put it to use. The principle remains the same no matter what position you assume: The wider your base of support, the less chance you have of losing your footing.

Slow, Slower, Slowest

True, Parkinson's disease slows people down. The very essence of the disorder is slowness. At the same time, PD also produces a kind of agitation in some patients, a feeling of hurry and urgent necessity. This reaction, needless to say, profits no one. It is better to simply slow down. Take it a step at a time; do whatever it is you are doing methodically, unhurriedly, without giving in to pressure. The more purposeful a movement is, the less likely it is to produce disequilibrium, and the less likely you are to fall. Slower is better for us all.

Strive to Keep an Upright Posture

Over time many PD people come to display a stooped posture with their head and shoulders bent forward and their chin tending toward the chest. But unlike certain other neurological ailments, patients are not helplessly locked into this position. There is simply a strong tendency to assume it. With effort it can usually be overcome.

A good exercise against this tendency is to stand in a doorway and prop your back tightly against the doorjamb. When properly lined up the doorjamb should touch the back of your head, neck, shoulder blades, the space between the small of the back, your buttocks, the backs of your knees, calves, and heels.

Remain in this position for several minutes, letting your body relearn its proper carriage. Think the posture out carefully to yourself: Where is my head now? Where is my back? Where are my heels? Take a mental picture of how you are standing. This position mimics the way you should stand all the time.

Now walk around the room for several minutes, then return to the doorway and check your posture. How much have you started to lean again?

Repeat this exercise whenever you can, each time trying to keep your spine as straight as possible. During the rest of the day use the mental photographs you have taken as a check against stooping. Frequent practice will help.

Caregivers can be a boon in this area by exhorting patients to stand upright during the course of the day. Caregivers can call attention to stooping when it occurs—patients are often unaware they are doing it. Or they can deliver gentle reminders to "do the doorjamb exercise" or "think of the doorjamb" whenever stooping becomes apparent.

More Tips for Maintaining Balance and Avoiding Falls

• Some people find their ambulatory self-confidence is improved by carrying something in their hands when they walk. The help object seems to act as a kind of ballast or counterweight against the tendency toward unsteadiness. A cane is perhaps the most useful piece of equipment for this purpose, though any portable item such as an umbrella, briefcase, or purse can help. There are even reports that commercial wrist and ankle weights help improve steadiness. Try them.

• Be careful of losing too much weight. PD people have a tendency to become thin, and with pounds go the vitality and muscle strength necessary to keep the legs steady. Loss of weight also attenuates the layers of fat that surround the hips, arms, legs, and shoulders, thus reducing one's natural padding should a fall occur.

• The receptors in the muscles and joints that monitor one's sense of position, space, and movement sometimes go out of whack in PD people and provide false readings on how short, how long, or how high things really are in one's surroundings. These sensory readings may be only slightly off, but this small discrepancy is all that's needed to discourage the feet from raising as high as they should when negotiating a lamp cord or a child's toy in the middle of the room. Exaggerate your steps. Raise your feet an inch higher and longer when you step over things. This extra effort will take up the slack made by errors in spacial judgment.

• If you have stairs in your home memorize the number of steps on each flight. Then count them out as you climb or descend. This trick will help you avoid tripping on those "extra" steps that seem to come out of nowhere at the bottom and top of landings.

• Look straight ahead when you walk, not down at the floor. Keeping your eyes cast downward pulls the rest of the body with it, the perfect setup for a fall.

• Try walking around the house barefoot. Patients report that the traction and added grip on rugs and smooth surfaces helps improve their footing.

• If you do fall, don't fight it. Simply allow your body to go limp, stay relaxed, and just sort of sink to the ground and roll with the momentum, keeping your arms in close to your body as you do. The more you flounder and flail against the downward movement, the greater will be your chances of getting hurt.

FREEZING

One of the most unpleasant side effects of the on/off syndrome is freezing. When this event occurs the feet simply stop moving. They refuse to respond, as if rooted to the floor. It can happen anywhere, anytime. Patients may find themselves paralyzed in front of a doorway, or in a bathroom incapable of getting out of the tub, or worst of all, halted helplessly in the middle of a busy street. Innumerable variations exist on the theme.

Moments of freezing tend to occur when too many things are demanded of a person at one time, or when the person's senses are overloaded with impressions—but not always. Freezing can also come for no apparent reason, and when it does the person must be prepared.

When Freezing Occurs Relax, Don't Panic

If you suddenly find yourself freezing up, keep your cool. Anxiety will makes things worse, not better. The best thing to do is simply to relax. If possible, sit down. Lean on something. Never castigate yourself for being unable to move—it will make things worse. Take a deep breath or two and sit quietly. Chances are the spell will be broken soon and you will be free to go on your way.

Getting Through Those Doorways

For reasons not entirely understood, PD people sometimes freeze when they are about to walk through a doorway. Confusing visual input stymies some patients, we know, and the narrowness of the door apparently bewilders those parts of the brain that process such information. There are several things you can do:

1. If you get stuck in a doorway simply stop and wait several minutes for the freezing to pass. It will.
2. If you are in a hurry sink slowly to your knees and crawl through the door. Obviously this is a maneuver you will wish to do at home only; and be aware that wall-to-wall carpeting guarantees a far easier time of it than wooden or tile floors.
3. A final trick is to cover your eyes. This action relieves the brain of threatening visual imagery and allows you to walk straight ahead without further trouble.

Let Others Help

If you freeze and cannot get unstuck, ask a friend, caregiver, or passer-by to help you in the following way: The caregiver should stand behind the patient, making sure that the patient's legs are set wide apart, and that his or her body is squared off and facing straight ahead. The caregiver informs the patient what is about to happen, then places his or her hands on the patient's shoulders and with a gentle rhythm starts to rock the person from side to side, then forward and backward. The caregiver counts out loud with each repetition: "One, two, three, four. . . ."

After building up momentum with this rhythmical swaying the caregiver gives the patient a gentle shove, being careful not to push too hard. The rocking movements will, as it were, warm the patient up and activate the parts of the brain responsible for ambulation. Patients can usually take it on their own from here.

Create Your Own Forward Momentum

Patients can also perform the same movements for themselves. Hold onto a nearby support. Slowly rock from side to side or forward and backward, gradually increasing the speed. After a short time you will feel looser and more energized. Now, still swaying rhythmically, start to march in place. Alternate your steps, right, left, right, left, building up to a brisk walk. Count out loud: "One, two, three, four; one, two, three, four." Once your legs are pumping and your rhythm is established, you should be able to step forward on your own.

Lay Out Visual Guidelines from Room to Room

It is the experience of many PD people that indicator markers arranged on the floor from room to room can help prevent freezing. A simple variety can be made with a length of white string. Lay it out on the floor from, say, the bedroom to the bathroom. When you get up at night the string will serve as a guide.

Why such a technique should discourage freezing is a mystery, but it does seem to work. Floor pathways can also be made with glow-in-the-dark tape.

FOUR SPECIAL MOVEMENT PROBLEMS

Getting Up from a Chair

Place your buttocks as far forward on the chair seat as they will comfortably go. Position yourself so that the backs of your legs are touching the legs of the chair and your body is leaning forward. This position is a crucial one. Spread your legs 8 to 10 inches apart. Grip the edges of the chair or hold the chair arms (armless chairs are usually easier for PD people). Rock back and forth several times to build up momentum, then, leading with your head, push yourself up and out into a standing position with one uninterrupted motion. Once you are up, assume a wide, firm base beneath your feet. Make sure you feel steady before attempting to walk.

You will find that deep cushions on sofas and easy chairs are more difficult to rise from than the harder surfaces of a wooden or metal stool; and high seats are easier to get out of than low ones. Some people raise the legs of their chairs an inch or two with wooden blocks or leg extenders. Special orthopedic equipment is available for this purpose from health supply stores.

To sit down, stand in front of the chair with your buttocks near the front of the seat and your legs as close to the chair legs as possible. Supporting yourself with your arms, ease yourself down in one slow, continuous motion. Keep your back as straight as possible as you go and make sure your body is well centered in relation to the chair.

Getting Out of a Car

Open the car door as wide as it will go. Rock slowly from side to side several times to build up steam. Then, gripping the dashboard or door handle, pivot your body one-half turn toward the door and push yourself up and out.

The most difficult part of this manipulation is, of course, the pivot, with all the many coordinated movements it demands. To make it easier, patients sometimes place a plastic bag beneath them on the car seat, taking advantage of its slick surface to make the turn smoother and less resistant. For those who don't wish to have plastic bags decorating their front seats, a piece of silk or any glossy, slippery material will do.

Getting Out of Bed

Getting out of bed in the morning is no easy matter for PD people. Deprived of medication for eight or nine hours, rigidity and bradykinesia have set in. Where are the tops of the covers? the PD person asks. Will my fingers be strong enough to grip them? Will

I have enough strength to untangle myself from the sheets and to lift the covers? Can I make it up to a sitting position on the side of the bed? Once I get there, will I be able to stand?

Thus, a special method for getting out of bed:

1. Lie flat on your back with your legs together.
2. Bend your knees to your chest.
3. Rock from side to side several times. (You can also build up momentum by swinging your arms back and forth across your chest three or four times.)
4. Using your backside as a pivot, in one continuous motion turn and roll over to a sitting position at the edge of the bed.
5. Note that some patients roll better to the right, some to the left. Find out which direction is best and then sleep on the side of the bed that allows the better roll. A spring mattress (as opposed to one made of foam rubber) will be especially helpful for this technique.

Sometimes patients are not able to roll over on their own no matter what turning technique they use. One couple solved this problem by tying one end of a smooth-surfaced cord to a window frame and the other to the bedstead. In the middle of the night when the woman needs to change her position she grabs the rope and uses it as a support to turn herself.

Couples have also discovered that positioning their bed next to a wall turns the wall into a fulcrum to push off from when rolling over. Others report that blanket supports keep the legs free of heavy blankets and make turning easier.

For people who have special difficulty getting out of bed it is imperative that a well-installed railing or grip surface be kept near the bed. Some patients, for example, sleep in beds that have a hospital-style half-railing mounted on the side. Others position a solid, heavy piece of furniture nearby to grip. Still others use beds that can be electronically raised and lowered. An overhead trapeze can also be used to pull oneself up, and is available from most orthopedic supply stores (see Chapter 14).

Carl D. has difficulty pushing off from his mattress, so he and his wife, Mary Jane, constructed a special post for the purpose that, with appropriate modifications, can be fitted to most beds. Here are the plans as drafted by Mary Jane:

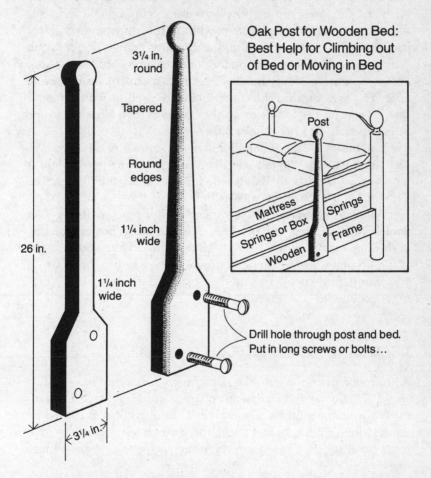

3¼ in. round

Tapered

Round edges

1¼ inch wide

26 in.

1¼ inch wide

3¼ in.

Oak Post for Wooden Bed: Best Help for Climbing out of Bed or Moving in Bed

Post

Mattress

Springs or Box

Wooden

Springs

Frame

Drill hole through post and bed. Put in long screws or bolts…

A last useful trick for getting out of bed in the morning and rolling over at night is to use satin sheets for easy sliding instead of sheets made of flannel or percale. Silk pajamas and nightgowns can be used for the same purpose.

Walking Up Stairs

First, be sure that stair safety in the patient's environment is maintained. See to it that the bannister is in good working order and that it is solidly embedded into the wall. Double railings, one on each side, are recommended by some occupational therapists, though going up and down stairs with both arms extended places patients in an awkward position and many people prefer single railings only. Rubber treads on the stairs are excellent for traction, and extra thick padding under the stair carpet protects in case of falls. The area around the stairs should be well lit with no loose scatter rugs on the treads or on the landings. See Chapter 14 for more on stair and household safety.

The basic rule for going up and down stairs is to do it *slowly*—one step at a time, literally and figuratively. Some people find it is easier to keep both hands on the railing as they ascend or descend, and to face the wall as they go. If this works, fine.

What if one freezes on the stairs? Don't fight it. Relax. Get your bearings. Then very carefully sink to a sitting position on one of the steps and wait for the off period to pass. Then continue on. If the off period is persistent, continue up the rest of the stairs on your hands and knees. This method can be difficult, and is recommended only as a last resort.

DEALING WITH DYSKINESIA

As one doctor remarked, "Dyskinesia is a separate disease all its own." Characterized by uncontrolled and disorganized involuntary movements of the arms, legs, face, and trunk, it is caused by medication, not by the PD itself, and as such can usually be kept under control by a physician. Here are a few tips that will also help:

• When dyskinesia becomes particularly troublesome, try taking a brisk ten- or fifteen-minute walk. Physical movement helps rid the body of the excess energy that dyskinesia thrives on, and it has an overall relaxing effect.

• A useful antidote for dyskinesia is exercise. Try following the routines outlined in Chapter 11. Stretches are particularly important in this regard. Sometimes a few minutes of brisk physical activity will also do the trick.

• If your arms are dyskinetic a trick that sometimes works is to hold them out in front of you, open and close your hands several times, then alternately tighten and loosen your arm muscles five or ten times in a row. When finished, drop your arms to your sides and relax them as completely as possible.

• For people on Sinemet, dyskinesia tends to come on with special intensity in the first few minutes after the medicine starts to work. Thus, plan your day with this fact in mind, keeping periods of the day when the medicine "clicks in" free from demanding duties.

IMPROVING YOUR HANDWRITING

A frequent first symptom heralding the onset of Parkinson's disease is a change in handwriting. Where words once flowed undeviatingly across the page, now lines of script display a crunched-up, claustrophobic appearance, tending to become increasingly smaller as they run from left to right.

While afflicted handwriting is indeed a disadvantage for people who prefer the pen over the typewriter or word processor, there are several tricks that will help you get your penmanship back on a relatively even keel.

Raise Your Hand Above Your Head
When You Are About to Write

If you are having difficulty holding a pen or keeping your letters steady, slowly raise your writing hand above your head. Hold it there for ten to fifteen seconds, giving your arm plenty of extension and stretching your fingers out as far as they will go. Then try again. You'll be surprised at the results. This sleek tip of Libby

Fine's, exercise leader of the Englewood, New Jersey, Parkinson's group, is remarkably simple yet has proven highly effective for many people.

Roll Your Hands

If your hands tend to cramp and you are having a difficult time getting pen to paper (or performing any manual task), take a cardboard mailing tube, place it on your lap, and roll it back and forth with your hands for several minutes. This rolling action will stimulate the circulation in your hands, wrists, and thighs and will have a loosening-up effect on the fingers.

Pause in Between Word Groups as You Write

The cramped appearance of handwriting can be helped by this method: Instead of trying to produce a line of script in a single unbroken movement of the pen, write a few words, stop, shift your hand a quarter inch to the right, and continue on. Make this shift every three or four words in a line.

Write on Lined Paper

PD people often do not realize how small and indistinguishable their handwriting appears to others. Paper with ruled lines will help, serving as a spacing guide, forcing the writer to produce penmanship of uniform size and preventing the words from trailing off or decreasing in size at the end of the line.

Print, Don't Write

The flowing, connected quality of script may look beautiful on the page but it can lend itself to intricate tangles for PD patients. Bold printed letters are simpler to work with and easier to write—and read. Whenever you can, print.

DEALING WITH SLEEP PROBLEMS

Sleep problems are a common side effect of Parkinson's disease and medications. In one study as many as 40 percent of PD patients reported some degree of difficulty falling asleep and staying asleep. They complained of exhaustion during the day, fitfulness at night, shortened sleep duration, and general restlessness during the nocturnal hours.[1] Such problems are especially unfortunate when you consider that during sleep the dopamine-producing cells that have managed to survive in a PD patient's brain are at their most active, manufacturing and storing dopamine. The more one's sleep is interrupted, the less these cells produce, and the worse a person's symptoms will be the next day.

Take Care of the Ordinary Sleep Essentials First

Start by recalling the eight major causes of poor sleep:

1. Caffeine stimulation (too much coffee, tea, soft drinks, use of over-the-counter preparations to prevent drowsiness)
2. Lack of daily activity and/or exercise
3. Uncomfortable sleeping conditions: noise in the bedroom, excess light, temperature too hot or cold, unaccommodating bed, hard pillow, itchy night clothes
4. Napping for long periods during the day, or sleeping too late in the morning
5. Excessive drinking of alcoholic beverages
6. Side effects of medication
7. Worry, mental overstimulation, anxiety
8. Full or weak bladder

With the above facts in mind, make a thorough check of your sleeping accommodations. Be sure your mattress is comfortable, your room temperature is pleasant, your pillow is the right degree of softness, and your night clothes are unbinding. Be sure no raucous noises or bright lights are around to bother you (if they are, sleep masks or ear plugs may help).

If your spouse snores or disturbs your sleep in any way, consider moving into a separate bed or, if necessary, a separate room. A king-sized mattress may help if your spouse tosses and turns.

Have a snack before you turn in, especially something with calcium in it like a glass of warm milk. Or conversely, don't eat and drink at all if a full bladder wakes you up. Try elevating your feet several inches when you sleep.

Falling asleep to soft music or relaxation tapes works for some people. But be careful: Studies have found that low droning noises such as air conditioners or even radios can interfere with REM (rapid eye movement) sleep and disturb sleep patterns.

Lambs wool undersheets have been touted as improving sleep quality, though nothing is proven along these lines. Don't, however, use too many blankets. Their weight can be subliminally disturbing. Electric blankets are light and put minimal pressure on the legs. Their dry, penetrating heat is soothing for some people, bothersome for others.

Determine the conditions that help you sleep best and stick to them. Every little improvement helps.

Don't Forget to Exercise

Our bodies were made to be active. When they become too passive or sedentary, restlessness and malaise set in. Thus, at least part of your day must be dedicated to physical activity if you wish to sleep well at night. Calisthenics are excellent for this purpose, as are walks, swimming, exercise machines, and any physical stimulation that stretches the muscles and raises the heartbeat.

To maximize the value of exercise it is best to do it in the morning or the middle of the day, not before going to bed. One of the most critical factors in getting to sleep is body temperature. If it is dropping at bedtime, you will have an easy time falling asleep. If it is going up, difficulties may ensue. Exercise raises the body's metabolic rate for several hours at a time and also the body's temperature. After five or six hours, the metabolism slows down again and the temperature drops accordingly. Thus, exercise at least five or six hours before you go to sleep. Patients who are habituated to hot baths or showers at night should also be warned. Hot baths raise body temperature and may interfere with sleep. Lukewarm baths are equally relaxing, but have a negligible effect on the body's thermostat.

Fine-Tune Your Medications

Sinemet and, according to some patients, Eldepryl, have a tendency to interfere with sleep. Patients can sometimes get around these difficulties by taking their last dose of medication four or five hours before sleep. There are no definites here though, since after a four- or five-hour doseless period people may experience increased general symptoms that interfere with getting to sleep. Perhaps simply cutting down on the last dose of the day by half will do, or by a quarter. Each person reacts differently to medication and each must find the combinations that work best.

Note further that anticholinergic drugs (including the antihistamines) have a natural sleep-inducing effect and can be used as a mild sleeping potion. Beware, however, of taking over-the-counter sleep medications with anticholinergics. Their ingredients, mainly the scopolamine, are similar to those in the anticholinergics and an overload can cause anticholinergic poisoning.

What to Do About Cramps

Some patients are awakened at night by muscle spasms that cause sudden tightening sensations in the legs. If this problem persists tell your doctor. He or she will probably prescribe quinine or a similar medication. Meanwhile, when medication is not immediately available you may find relief by:

- Elevating your legs
- Massaging your legs (or better, having them massaged)

- Applying heat packs
- Pounding or applying percussion up and down your legs
- Brisk walking and stretching

More Tips for Good Sleep

- Walks to the bathroom at 3 A.M. can be dangerous business, especially if you suffer from balance problems. They can also wake you up for the rest of the night. A plastic urinal (available at any pharmacy) kept by the bedside will eliminate this problem. Portable urinals are available for women as well as for men.
- Refrain from drinking liquids after dinner. The less fluid there is in your bladder at bedtime, the less chance you have of waking up to urinate during the night.
- Since protein interferes with the digestion of Sinemet and slows its transport to the brain, take your regular dose of Sinemet at night and then eat a meal heavy of protein. It will slow the dopaminergic effect of the drug just enough to allow you to fall asleep but not enough to prevent the drug from working.
- Try old-time natural remedies for sleep enhancement. The most effective ones include a glass of hot milk with honey; a rubdown; several handfuls of lettuce (lettuce has opium in it); herb teas (camomile, scullcap, valerian root, hops); rubbing the inside of your wrists with a circular motion, a minute on each wrist—keep repeating (this is the latest method from Scandinavia); counting sheep (or a better variation: imagine a blackboard with the number 10 written on it. Picture a hand erasing the 10 and writing a 9, then erasing the 9 and writing an 8, and so on down to zero. Run through this sequence several times).

GETTING AROUND: BECOME SELECTIVE
ABOUT WHEN, WHERE, AND HOW

PD is full of contradictions. Patients must get out of the house frequently if they wish to maintain their full range of physical and mental acuity. But at times the outside world can become complex and overdemanding; it can tax one's limits with too many impressions and too many decisions. Thus, PD people must remain selective about where they go, and when, and how they get there. It is truly "life in the slow lane," as one patient termed living with PD.

If you have a general idea of when your on and off periods come—and these, as you know, depend largely on your medication—schedule your time accordingly so that you do your shopping, phone calling, driving, and visiting during the best times of day and keep the off periods for rest. For shopping, fewer people are in the supermarkets and malls during the morning hours. Schedule accordingly. If you drive, keep off the roads during peak traffic hours. Make all pickups and deliveries between 10 A.M. and 3 P.M. when traffic flow is contained. If you are going to take a bus or subway, travel during the off hours.

During Christmas time it may be wise to send a relative out to do your shopping, or you may wish to shop by mail. If you live in a city and enjoy excursions, pick the times of day when streets and parks are least populated. If you walk to work consider taking a longer but less crowded route to get there.

In social situations, be careful of conversing with several people at once. Keep each conversation separate and one-on-one. Doing more than one thing at a time in a social situation can become confusing. Pick relatively quiet, uncrowded places to do your socializing: a local restaurant or a neighborhood social center. You will probably feel better associating with people you already know. New situations tend to be intimidating for many PD people.

About Driving

Should you drive or shouldn't you drive? This can be a thorny issue and one that often becomes a bone of contention in the family household. The caregiver, afraid for the patient's safety (and perhaps for his or her own), seems to notice every driving error the patient makes, and may trot out a laundry list of grievances whenever the topic is discussed.

PD people, on the other hand, treasure their driving privilege. It is a sign of competency, an indication that they still have some control over their already shrunken world. To take this privilege away may be tantamount to telling patients that they are now invalids. Driving is a symbol of independence and self-reliance.

The choice must rest with the patient. *But,* at the same time, the patient should first be informed about the following 5 facts:

1. Parkinson's disease detracts from a person's driving abilities. PD patients take longer to hit the brake—much longer. They don't see as well out the rear-view mirror or from the side. The chances exist of their hands locking on the wheel or of not being able to turn the wheel properly. The more one's condition progresses, the poorer one's driving skills become. And the greater the chances are of hurting oneself and others. A serious tremor, vision deficits, freezing, slowness of reaction time, stiffness of the wrists and braking foot, difficulties in spacial perception, and all the other typical symptoms of Parkinson's disease can, and almost inevitably do, contribute to decreased driving skills.

2. In certain states, if a PD driver gets into an accident, and it can be proven that it was caused by the driver's neurological debility, that person may be liable to legal action.

3. In some states, automobile insurance may be raised considerably if a driver suffers from a neurological disease.

4. If you have any doubts about your motoring skills many hospitals offer driver evaluation courses. Examiners will test reflexes, sight and hearing, reaction time, hand-to-eye coordination, and other physical skills essential for alert driving. The hospital will then give testees a full report and suggest any modifications that they determine are necessary. They will also advise *against* driving if they feel the person's test scores are too low.

5. For the caregiver especially, if the PD person's driving skills are dangerously below par and if the patient stubbornly refuses to give up the wheel, even after several near-misses, here is a strategy that almost always works. Ask your doctor to tell the patient that his or her health and coordination no longer meet the standards of highway safety, and that it is strongly "suggested" he or she give up their driver's license. Coming from an authority figure such as the family physician, this decree will carry weight, as opposed to when it comes from a caregiver or family member who often find their protests dismissed out of hand.

Here are some comments made by patients and caregivers concerning the driving problem:

Patient: Most people can tell when it's time to stop driving. You feel it, it's a sixth sense. I felt that I would be a hazard so I stopped.

Caregiver: I told her, "Do you want to become a statistic?" I asked her, "Do you want to cause an accident? Do you want to hit a child or an old lady with a cane?"

Patient: I stopped driving when four or five people told me my driving was becoming dangerous. I didn't even realize it but I was weaving all over the road. Sometimes you have to listen to others.

Caregiver: I let Walter drive cause he can still handle the wheel well. I feel that as long as he seems competent why make a fuss. Only once did he make a mistake due to his Parkinson's disease. His tremor acted up and we went too far to the right. Since then he's become extra careful.

Patient: I feel comfortable when my brother is in the car with me, or a friend. I drive, but only if someone else is with me to take over should there be trouble, should I go off (which hasn't happened yet while I'm driving) or should I get very tired (this has).

Caregiver: I encourage Joyce to drive on the back roads during the off hours of the day. She goes short distances to the supermarket and pet store. I do *not* allow her to drive on the superhighways or in high traffic.

Tips for Travelers

When Parkinson's patients travel for business or leisure they face a number of specialized problems that can make their trip less than pleasurable. As a hedge against potential difficulty on the road or in the air, make as many compensatory plans and arrangements as possible beforehand to smooth the way.

For example, reserve bus, train, or airline tickets well in advance. If you know a good travel agent all arrangements can be made over the phone. Book a trip that departs at a time of day, week, and month when the airports or terminals are least crowded (5:00 P.M. is the busiest hour of the day; Friday, Saturday, and Sunday are the busiest days of the week; June to September are the most traveled times of year). Avoid traveling at holiday time if you possibly can.

Enquire about getting roomy bulkhead seating in the front of the plane when traveling by air. Most airlines reserve these seats for handicapped people and for families traveling with children. Go nonstop if you can; it will mean less time cooped up in the flight cabin, and you won't have to face the strain of changing planes. If you suffer from bladder difficulties reserve your chair on the aisle so you can get to the restrooms with a minimum of difficulty. When booking you can also, if necessary, arrange to be met at both airports by a porter with a wheelchair. Confirm these arrangements the day before you leave.

Canvas suitcases are especially light and portable. Make sure your suitcase has wheels. Take two sets of medication and separate them when you pack in case one gets lost. That is, tuck one set into your carry-on luggage, and another in your heavier luggage. Carry-on luggage should be minimal.

Dress comfortably when on a plane. Scientists now know that loose-fitting clothes and nonbinding shoes help reduce jet lag. Drink plenty of fluids as well: four or five glasses of water or juice at the minimum. The liquid will fight jet lag and will keep you hydrated. If you are traveling alone make sure you have identification on your person stating that you are a Parkinson's person and giving directions for any specific medical needs you may have in case of an accident or emergency.

THE SEX QUESTION

Except for exceptional cases, patients find that their sexual functions are relatively unaffected by Parkinson's disease. Complaints of impotency or frigidity are rare, at least in the beginning, and these are usually due to medications or depression rather than to the disease itself.

A small percentage of male patients react to Sinemet with an *increase* in erections, some to the point of developing priapism. But not many. Most reports of increased sexual activity have less to do with the mythical aphrodisiac qualities of L-dopa than with the simple fact that any improvement in overall body functioning tends to increase sexual vitality as well.

However, over the years the sexual urge does seem to diminish in PD patients. As time passes the patient becomes imperceptibly less interested, less focused on sex. Part of this reaction is due to the aging process itself, part to psychological complications, and part to the fact that one does, after all, suffer from a chronic neurological disease and chronic diseases take their toll on every part of the body. Sexuality is maintained in the human organism by a delicate combination of good physical health and psychological well-being. In times of danger or trouble it is, along with appetite, the first of the physical functions to shut down. Imagine then over the long run what a toll the psychophysical afflictions of PD must take on the already sensitive libido.

Still in all, PD is not the type of ailment that attacks the sexual function directly or that embarrasses one's potency. Most couples enjoy a relatively normal sex life, though in many cases it must be reduced in duration, frequency, and liveliness. Rigidity and bradykinesia can, moreover, create problems in body logistics, especially in the ability to thrust and maintain rhythmical movements. Creative couples will come up with their own accommodations to these difficulties as they occur.

When and if sexual dysfunctions such as impotence do appear, this development is usually due to medications, specifically tranquilizers and anticholinergics. Consult with your physician. Dryness on the woman's part may be a result of many possible influences and is not cause for alarm. Lubricating creams and jellies usually solve the problem.

Patients and caregivers offer the following experiences:

Patient: I have no lack of desire. I just can't move very well when I do it. Listen, I can't get out of bed in the morning, how the hell do you expect me to be Don Juan? We manage. Want the secret? Letting my wife stay on the top and do the work. Not bad for an old man!

Caregiver: We had a few sexual problems at first but my husband wouldn't talk to the doctor about them. I finally went myself and told him. The doctor had several suggestions. Make love during the "on" periods. Use lubricating cream. They were good. I passed them onto my husband.

Patient: In the beginning when I was diagnosed we had no problems sexually. As time has passed we've developed a few. I have become dry sometimes and can't move around enough to please my husband. He, in return, has become impotent with (I guess) loss of desire due to my pathetic performances in bed. Sex was once very important to us. Now it's not. It just happens that way.

Patient: The word that comes to mind is *compensation*. Our sexual life is not what it used to be but it's still pretty good because instead of letting the losses get us down we've worked to make the best of what we've got. We've also figured out things that compensate for the losses. I can't move as well as I could. My wife does most of it now. I have trouble keeping time so she does most of that. If I have to stop in the middle of the act and rest we lie there and just talk. That's nice. Almost as nice as the sex. We're both happy with the way it is and grateful that we can still enjoy one another.

Patient: Our love life revolves around my "on" periods. We try to plan our times to coincide with them. When I'm "on" sex isn't bad, everything considered. When I'm "off" sex is out of the question.

Caregiver: Like a lot of things with Parkinson's disease, you just have to accept your sexual losses along with the other losses. We are all born to die and we are all born to be sick at some time in our lives. We all sow our wild oats and then later pay the piper. That's just how it is. That's the cycle of life. Now my wife and I are paying the piper. When we can accept this fact our days are calm and we are happy. Acceptance is the antidote to all disease and to every misfortune. When you have acceptance nothing in the world can hurt you. You become free.

FATIGUE

Whenever PD people move they must, as it were, carry the added weight of rigidity and tremor along with them. These extra burdens work the muscles mercilessly from hour to hour, and place extra strain on the joints. Imagine how much energy it must take to simply keep a shaking limb in motion for ten or twelve hours straight. Imagine the effort it takes in the muscles to keep the arms or the legs tight and tense for so long a time. By the end of the day patients have done double duty. They have coped with the exigencies of ordinary living, and they have endured the energy-sapping debilities of PD.

Ways in which this fatigue level can be reduced include the following:

• Exercise, exercise, exercise. Nothing feeds fatigue like inactivity. Sleeping breeds more sleeping. Constant lying down breeds the need to lie down some more. Wise patients keep at least part of their days reserved for exercise and effort. They know that activity gives them energy. That's how it works; that's where energy comes from.

• In later stages of PD some patients find they must lie down for long periods of the day and must husband their energies carefully, keeping busy in the morning, say, because they know that by afternoon exhaustion will set in. Thus, plan your day with the ups and downs in mind. Observe when your best periods are and get your heavy-duty work in at this time. Plan your day so that necessary social obligations and work activities are scheduled accordingly. Reserve the off times for rest.

• Try various relaxation alternatives. Consider learning meditation techniques. Biofeedback has helped PD patients deal with fatigue and has helped them overcome bothersome minor irritations like headaches and sore backs. Do-it-yourself books on self-hypnosis and relaxation are valuable. Sources that deal in relaxation and tension-reducing resources include:

> Relaxation tapes and guided imagery with music; 30-minute cassette tales engineered for relaxation at bedtime: Guidance System, Gwynedd Plaza II, Suite 301, Spring House, PA 19477

> The "Self-Care Catalog" offers many relaxation and stress-reduction materials: Self-Care Catalog, P.O. Box 999, Pt. Reyes, CA 94956

> Sleep-inducing self-hypnosis tapes: B. K. Enterprises, 9478 Olympic Blvd., P.O. Box 6248, Beverly Hills, CA 90212

A variety of materials designed to relieve stress and help relaxation: Conscious Living Foundation, P.O. Box 9, Drain, OR 97435

A company that specializes in books and tapes dedicated to relaxation: New Harbinger Publications, 2200 Adeline, Suite 305, Oakland, CA 94607

NOTE

1. J. Thomas Hutton and Raye Lynne Dippel, *Caring for the Parkinson Patient* (Buffalo, New York: Prometheus Books, 1989), 109.

13

Managing 2:
More Hints

EATING

When a healthy person eats dinner a sequence of complex muscular and salivary activities takes place in his or her mouth that is synchronized in a remarkably coordinated manner. Like a symphony orchestra the various organs—saliva glands, jaws and teeth, tongue, lips, epiglottis, muscles of the mouth and throat—all make their contribution at exactly the precise moment in order to create chewing and swallowing harmony. Even a second's delay will throw the whole process off, with coughing, choking, and possible aspiration of food into the lungs as the result.

Now the symptoms of PD, especially bradykinesia and rigidity, can affect any part of the body, the mouth and swallowing apparatus included. When this occurs how does it impact the eating process?

In several ways. For one, when food is eaten it must be chewed to make it soft and digestible. But if the large jaw muscles are weakened, mastication will become difficult and large chunks of food will go unprocessed. Swallowing is done in three steps. First, the tongue forms the food into a *bolus* or compact mass and pushes it against the soft palate in the back of the throat, causing the swallowing reflex to trigger. But if the tongue is weak and unresponsive the food may never reach its destination. Second, the muscles of the throat move the food down to the esophagus. But if these muscles are not working properly food becomes lodged in place. Finally, food passes into the esophagus and on to the stomach. Here digestion difficulties can occur.

Statistically speaking, approximately half of all PD patients develop problems somewhere along the line in this chewing-swallowing chain. In many cases they need help, and in most instances this help can be given. A majority of the information that follows comes from licensed speech therapists and rehabilitation specialists. Special thanks go to speech language pathologists Jane Goldberg and Ellen Greenfield, members of the Nyack Hospital Rehabilitation Department staff, for their information, involvement, and concern.

The Careful Eater

You will know if you are having swallowing problems. They are self-evident. Swallowing becomes increasingly difficult and, it seems, you must chew forever just to get a single bite of food down. Excessive coughing and salivation are also tip-offs, as is food that sticks to your tongue and refuses to move to the back of the throat no matter how hard you try to force it. If you have trouble in any of these departments, the first thing you can do is to become selective about what foods you eat and how you eat them.

Avoid Thin Liquids

Observe how a dollop of mashed potatoes or a spoonful of applesauce sits stolidly on your tongue, and how easily it is moved to the back of the throat when you swallow. It is because these foods are semisolids; for most PD people they pose no swallowing problems.

Thin liquids, on the other hand, flow quickly to the back of the throat without waiting to be helped along by the tongue. Here they confuse the swallowing mechanism that is already working a beat or two off its timing cycle. Coughing and choking usually result. To remedy this problem avoid drinking thin liquids with meals including:

coffee	soda	water
tea	grape juice	mineral water
broth	apple juice	milk

If you are going to drink liquids with your meal thicken them first. For instance, prepare creamy soups instead of broths. Load up on fruit nectars rather than watery juices. Drink yogurt shakes or eggnog rather than milk. Add gravy to watery foods to make them more consistent. Eat Jell-O or ice cream instead of sherbet.

In general, food must be cooked for long periods of time before it reaches the proper degree of thickness. Unfortunately, too much cooking reduces both flavor and nutritional content. You can overcome this problem by using a commercial additive product known as *Thick-It 2,* a flavorless modified fruit starch that may be added to any liquid and that instantly thickens it into an easily swallowable, semisolid mass. *Thick-It 2* can be ordered from the Milani Company toll-free at 800-333-0003. The Milani Company also makes an easily swallowable line of vitamins and mineral supplements.

Don't Mix Food Textures

Beware, for instance, of eating thin soup with pieces of rice added. With its sticky, granulated texture rice is one of the first foods patients find difficult to swallow, especially when it is served in combination with a watery broth. If you are preparing a creamy soup that contains meat chunks, grains, or potatoes, puree these foods first until they are consistent with the texture of the soup.

Be careful of drinking fluids with your meals. For example, suppose you are munching on some french fries and decide to wash them down with a sip of coffee. The sensory receptors of the mouth and throat are already working at a reduced capacity due to the disease and can barely manage to measure each food adequately as it comes along. Add a second or third texture and the whole mechanism goes awry. As a general axiom, PD patients with oral-motor problems should drink *after* meals, not with them.*

Semisolid Is Best

Semisolid portions of puddings, mashed potatoes, squash, and oatmeal are by far the easiest to handle. Be careful of dry crumbly items such as hard rolls, toast, bread crumbs, chunky peanut butter, crackers, and rice. These are more easily processed in the mouth and throat if gravy is added or if they are first dunked in a liquid. Find out which foods go down easiest for you, which foods can be improved by thickening or thinning, and which foods are the most troublesome to swallow. A number of eating problems can be resolved by using experience and common sense.

Eliminate Pocketing

Dry foods, especially crackers, toast, and sandwiches, tend to "pocket" in the mouth of those with swallowing disorders. Pocketing occurs when particles of food become lodged in the gums and inner cheeks, and then remain there, sometimes for hours, sometimes for days, until they cause choking or infection. If pocketing is a problem, be sure that (1) the patient drinks after every meal, (2) the patient's mouth is washed out frequently, and (3) the patient's diet consists mainly of moist, semisolid foods.

---

*Some patients, it should be added here for the record, who have problems transporting food to the back of the mouth due to lack of tongue precision, take liquids after each mouthful and report favorably on the matter. Taking liquids in this way is especially helpful for foods that tend to crumble or flake apart like muffins and dry bread.

Pace Yourself

Eat slowly and pause in between each bite. After you empty your mouth, swallow to make sure all is clear before taking in more food. Keep your mouth tightly closed while you chew.

Remember to swallow frequently while you are eating. Some patients place signs near the dinner table saying, "Remember to swallow." Caregivers can reinforce this message by reminding patients to chew thoroughly during the course of the meal.

Watch Your Posture

Keeping the back straight while you eat will make digestion and swallowing easier. Avoid allowing the head to fall backward—this closes the throat and extends an open invitation to choking. A straight-backed chair will also help; so will remaining seated upright for at least twenty minutes after eating.

If hunching is a problem a plate can be brought closer to the mouth by raising it with a telephone book or other support. Finally, never eat lying down. It increases the chances of choking a dozenfold.

Other Tips for Better Chewing and Swallowing

• If you are having difficulty swallowing try stimulating your throat with a thick hot or cold drink. Cold and hot liquids both heighten the sensitivity of the swallowing reflex and force it into activity. (To prevent choking, be sure your mouth is clear of foods before you drink.) In general, foods that are heated or cooled are processed better by the chewing mechanism than foods served at room temperature.

• If eating utensils cause you to gag, try placing the fork or spoon on the tip of your tongue and then slowly slide it from the front of the tongue to the back in a single gentle motion. Never suddenly plop a spoonful of food down on the back or middle part of the tongue.

• If pills cause choking, mixing them with applesauce, pureed fruit, and/or soft vegetables like pureed carrots will help make swallowing easier. If the puree is slightly warm this will help even more.

• Bedridden people are advised to stay awake for at least twenty to thirty minutes after eating a meal. This extra time allows the food to clear the esophagus and to digest properly, thus reducing the chances of regurgitation (and choking) during the night.

• Take small bites when you eat. Keep conversation to a minimum. Caregivers should never rush patients at the table. Let them take as much time as they need to comfortably finish their meals. Some patients are served the first course of the meal before others to provide them with a head start.

• Since people with swallowing disorders eat very slowly, try increasing the number of meals served during the day and decreasing the amount of food served at each.

• Patients occasionally discover that one side of their tongue is stronger and more sensitive than the other. If you find this to be true, place all food midway on the good part of the tongue and chew favoring this side. The middle and the back sections are best.

• Drinking fluids through a straw will help prevent choking. Straws act as a natural check gauge, allowing a limited, monitored quantity of substance to pass into the mouth at a time. Flexistraws are especially good for this purpose.

• Eat during "on" periods and be careful when "off." Make sure that food taken during off times is soft and chewable enough for the weakened swallowing reflex to handle.

• For advanced PD patients who tend to gag on water or thin liquids, taking liquids by the spoonful will get them down and will reduce choking.

• Remember to swallow as often as you can while you chew. Remind yourself of this continually.

• Every person in the patient's family should know how to perform the Heimlich maneuver in case choking does occur.

DROOLING AND DRY MOUTH

PD patients do not produce more saliva than nonparkinsonians. They simply swallow less frequently. This delay causes the saliva that would ordinarily be washed down to pool in the mouth. The accumulation ultimately leads to overflow.

Unfortunately, no one has come up with a foolproof solution for overcoming drooling. Anticholinergic drugs dry out the mouth and help reduce excess salivation. But patients report that they tend to drool despite the medication. Thus, a double, contradictory problem arises: drooling and parched mouth.

Though neither of these conditions can be entirely eliminated, there are things that will help. The following tips may reduce drooling:

• For people who maintain good control over their swallowing, chewing gum is a useful aid against excess salivation because it forces chewers to swallow every several minutes. When you chew gum it is practically impossible *not* to swallow. Those who find gum a nuisance will be pleased to discover that sour balls or commercial hard candies accomplish the same results. For persons with a natural health bent, a handful of flax seeds chewed every half hour or so reputedly helps tongue and mouth muscle agility.

• Whenever you can, remember to keep your head up and your posture straight. Leaning or stooping encourages drooling.

• Keep your mouth closed and your lips tightly together when you are not talking or eating. PD people have a tendency to let their jaw drop open, which invites dribbling.

• Before you are about to talk, swallow first, then proceed. This will eliminate dribbling and will prevent embarrassment during conversation.

• Consciously remind yourself to swallow. Do this on your own or have a caregiver do it for you. Even three or four extra swallows per hour will cut down substantially on saliva buildup.

• Some people rub a pungent lip balm over their mouth to act as a swallowing reminder. Every time they become aware of the slight burning sensation the salve produces, it triggers them to swallow.

• Breathe from your nose as much as possible. Mouth breathing encourages an open mouth; nose breathing encourages a closed mouth. Nose breathing is also better for your health.

• Place one or two drops of atropine eyedrops (0.5 percent) under your tongue to reduce saliva output. This trick seems to work for some people, though consulting with your doctor before trying it is recommended.[1]

The following tips may help dry mouth:

• Chewing gum or sucking on hard candies helps keep the mouth lubricated. Again, this suggestion is for those who are not at risk of choking.

• Nose breathing (as opposed to mouth breathing) helps prevent the mouth from becoming parched. Breathe through your nose when you are at home, watching TV, lying down, wherever. Nose breathing will force you to keep your mouth closed and your lips together.

• Avoid eating dry foods such as crackers, peanut butter, and potato chips. They stick to the throat and dry out the mucus membranes of the mouth.

• Stay adequately hydrated. Drinking five or six glasses of water a day will help, though be careful of liquids and foods that produce thirst such as sugared soda, spicy foods, peanuts, and salty snacks. PD people have a tendency to drink too little and to become dehydrated. One neuropsychologist at a local hospital advises spouses or caregivers to fill a large pitcher or 1-liter soda bottle with juice or water in the morning, and place it on the dining table with a written reminder to "Finish contents by the time I return home at 5:00." This technique works especially well for forgetful patients.

• Take a cotton swab, dip it in olive oil, and rub the inside of your mouth and throat with it. Repeat every hour or so.

• If you smoke, cut down; or better yet, stop. Smoking can be a major factor in drying out the mouth and causing gum problems. Note too that caffeine dries the mucus membranes of the nose and throat, and can also contribute to excessive mouth dryness.

• If your mouth becomes unbearably dry consult your physician. Chances are your medications are causing the problem, especially if you are taking anticholinergics. A change or modification in dosage will usually help.

• Artificial saliva products are available if the need arises. Check with your doctor on this one.

DIET

On the whole, diet does not seem to have a significant effect on a PD person's symptoms (with several possible exceptions that are discussed below), and patients are usually advised simply to eat a well-rounded, nutritious diet. Certainly the dietary factors discussed above such as consistency and texture of food are of more immediate concern, and in the long run are more likely to cause trouble.

At the same time, we are what we eat, and there are principles of nutrition that every parkinsonian should know. On an individual, anecdotal level many patients report interesting dietary side-trips that may be worth exploring. Let's have a look.

The Protein Question

The most significant dietary concern is the relationship between protein and PD medication. Studies conducted at the Yale University Department of Neurology and elsewhere indicate that for some patients dietary protein taken at the same time as Sinemet temporarily interferes with the absorption of the Sinemet and slows down its effects. This interference takes place in two parts of the body: in the digestive system, and then again in the circulation of the medication up to the brain. For some people excess protein intake exacerbates the on/off syndrome as well.

The reason for this reaction is explained by the fact that L-dopa is an amino acid and is processed by the body in the same way as any other food protein. When dietary protein and L-dopa enter the gut at the same time they end up competing with each other for absorption, and some of the L-dopa gets lost in the digestive process. The more protein that is taken in, the more it interferes with the medication.

For this reason many doctors suggest that patients avoid heavy-protein meals during the daytime hours, and/or that they take their protein at times that do not coincide with their pill-taking schedule. The Yale Parkinson's Clinic recommends a low-protein diet for breakfast and lunch, then a normal amount of protein at dinner.

Some researchers also suggest that patients eat less protein in general. One study made in 1976 concludes that 30 grams of protein a day for a person weighing 132 pounds is adequate. A person weighing 155 pounds should limit intake to around 35 grams of protein a day. A person weighing 170 pounds should take 39 grams a day, and a person weighing 200 pounds should be limited to 46 grams a day. Though these amounts are below the adult recommended dietary allowance (RDA), they come close enough to the minimum daily level to satisfy most people's needs.[2] Foods high in protein include meat of all kinds, fish, nuts, peanuts, peanut butter, dairy products, and soy, lima, kidney, and white beans. Foods with trace amounts of protein include fruits, cucumbers, herbs, leafy vegetables, soda, oils, jams, and jellies. Grains tend to be extremely low-protein foods.

Patients would also do well to consult with their physician, and if given the green light, to observe the protein-Sinemet balance in their own systems. Be aware though that many patients find that their protein and their Sinemet get along just fine, and that they have no trouble assimilating the two together. If you fall into this category, the protein question becomes merely academic.

VITAMINS

Some may help; some may hinder. Vitamin E, many patients have found, seems to have some beneficial effects. Being a free-radical antioxidant it theoretically serves as a protection for dopamine-producing cells and prevents them from being destroyed at too rapid a rate. Nothing is guaranteed here, and nothing has been proven. In fact, Dr. Roger Duvoisin remarks that his attempts to use vitamin E to relieve leg cramps had no effect whatsoever on testees.[3]

Be that as it may, many patients report good results from this substance and it can't hurt to try it. In moderation vitamin E is harmless, and it can be useful as a food supplement if nothing else. One capsule of 400 international units in the morning and one at bedtime is the recommended dose.

Other anecdotal reports tout vitamin C as a possible aid. Injections of B_{12} given by doctors are sometimes used to raise a patient's energy levels, though this one is conjectural. Salt tablets are taken by some people as a counterbalance to the low blood pressure caused by medications. According to some studies, the amino acid diphenylalanine has proven useful in combating depression. Do stay away from the L-phenylalanine form, however. It is reputed to make the symptoms of PD worse.

Finally, know that vitamin B_6, which is included in most multivitamin supplements, interferes with the action of pure L-dopa, breaking it down before it can get by the blood-brain barrier. When the L-dopa is mixed with an enzyme inhibitor such as carbidopa the problems disappear. Since very few people take straight L-dopa anymore, and since Sinemet has become the standard form of this drug, the danger of vitamin B_6 is no longer much of an issue.

WEIGHT AND APPETITE

Because several neurotransmitters, including dopamine, participate in the control of appetite, and because both dopamine and related agents such as serotonin and acetylcholine are affected by PD, patients often find their appetite reduced, sometimes drastically. Add difficulty swallowing and depression to this fact and we find that many PD people lose weight.

It is imperative that eating be kept up on a regular basis. Dramatic weight loss can weaken PD sufferers who need all the vigor they can get. If the loss becomes severe it will reduce immunity to disease as well. Likewise, avoid trying to put back lost pounds with sweets or massive servings of food. Just include more complex carbohydrates with meals, especially pastas, potatoes, cereals, and breads. If you have any questions concerning nutrition or appetite control, consult your physician and/or a nutritionist.

CONSTIPATION

While many PD medications cause constipation, other elements contribute to the problem also: stress, depression, poor eating habits, insufficient exercise, and low fluid intake. Plain common sense is often the best cure.

Modify Your Diet and Add Plenty of Fiber

Fiber is the nonmetabolized residue of plant tissue, the parts that pass through the body undigested and exit largely intact. You won't find this substance in meats, fish, or dairy products. Fiber comes exclusively from the plant kingdom, specifically from vegetables, fruits, grains, and nuts.

In the gut, fiber exerts a strong absorbent action, drawing local stores of water into the feces and swelling their size and weight. These stores add both bulk and softness to the stool and make it pass swiftly and easily through the digestive tract. Tests show that people who eat a high-fiber diet eliminate more frequently than those who don't. Their feces are larger and fuller, and more waste materials are excreted at each bowel movement. Apples, avocados, beets, bran, broccoli, cabbage, corn, green beans, grits, lentils, mangoes, parsnips, peas, prunes, potatoes in their skins, raspberries, rolled oats, and strawberries are all rich in dietary fiber.

Exercise Regularly

Inactivity leads directly to sluggish bowels. Stretches, lifts, and, if feasible, workouts on a bicycle machine will tone the gut and get the juices flowing. Three times a week is an acceptable number of workouts; once a day is best. When you get up in the morning run through a few stretching exercises to get your blood flowing and the gastrointestinal system working quickly. For exercise routines see Chapter 11.

The Laxative Question

Many members of the medical community regard laxatives with a dubious eye. These controversial substances easily become habit-forming. Many brands irritate the lining of the colon and overuse can cause constipation rather than cure it. Laxatives sap the vigor of the digestive system, and excessive intake can atrophy key digestive organs. In the end, the eliminative system loses its ability to function without the stimulation of a laxative chemical. Addiction is the result.

Nevertheless, the occasional use of laxatives may be a necessary evil, particularly if dietary methods prove ineffective. In such cases, begin with the most gentle variety, the so-called *bulk-forming laxatives*. These include:

Wheat bran

Oat bran (also good for lowering cholesterol, recent studies indicate)

Psyllium derivatives (Metamucil, Siblin, Konsyl, Mucilose)

Malt soup extract (Maltsupex)

Polycarbophil (Mitrolan tablets)

Take these preparations with plenty of water, and be careful not to mix them with aspirin. If you have any questions about combining laxatives with your PD medications consult your physician.

If bulk-forming laxatives fail to do the job, *stool softeners* such as Bu-Lax, D-S-S, Colace, and Laxinate may help, but take them only for one day, or two at most. *Lubricant laxatives* such as mineral oil are sometimes effective, though overuse will interfere with proper nutrient absorption (taking mineral oil at bedtime can occasionally cause elderly people to aspirate the oil from the stomach into the lungs). Suppositories work for some people. However, *saline laxatives* such as milk of magnesia and tartar salts can cause loss of important body salts and are not frequently recommended.

The most powerful of all laxatives are the *stimulant laxatives*. These act directly on the intestines, artificially speeding up the transit time food takes to move through the bowels. Drugs included in this category are:

Castor oil

Bile salts (Ox Bile Extract)

Bisacodyl (Cenalax, Fleet Bisacodyl, Ducolax, Bisco-Lax)

Cascara sagrada

Phenolphthalein (Ex-Lax, Feen-a-Mint, Phenolax)

Senna (Senexon, Senokot)

It is suggested that you take stimulant laxatives only as a last resort, and then only for a few days at most. They work too well: The bowels quickly become dependent on them if overused.

Other Help for Constipation

• Eat plenty of fruits, whole grains, and leafy vegetables, and stay away from too many refined carbohydrates such as polished rice, white sugar, and white bread. The majority of these foods have their fiber stripped from them and tend to lack body. Inside the digestive tract they move ponderously along, digesting slowly and failing to stimulate the lining of the gut in the way that high-fiber foods do.

• Eliminate constipation-producing foods such as chocolate, sweets, fatty meat, hot and spicy foods, and alcohol.

• If tolerated, add natural laxative foods to your diet. These include yogurt, rhubarb, bran products, pumpkin seeds, papaya juice, prunes, cabbage, prune juice, and flax seeds.

• Eat foods that ferment quickly in the gut such as sauerkraut, sauerkraut juice, cabbage juice, sourdough bread, and pickles. For some people the addition of sauerkraut alone will restore regularity.

• Drink plenty of liquids. This easy step is often neglected, but it can really help. When you get up in the morning, drink a glass of lukewarm water. During the day drink seven or eight glasses of water or juice, and stick to this regimen faithfully.

• Take a bowlful of wheat berries (available at health food stores), boil them in water until soft, and eat them with fruit every morning for breakfast. Do this for a month straight. Some people report wonderful results from this simple remedy.

SPEECH AND COMMUNICATION

Many of the muscle groups that cause eating and gagging disorders contribute to speech impairments as well. About half of all PD patients suffer from some problem in this area, and often a speech impairment is the first symptom of Parkinson's disease to appear. This disorder attacks the speaking mechanism from several sides at once, producing difficulties with volume as well as with phrasing, rhythm, and clarity. Typical speech impairment problems are:

- A tendency to slur words
- A tremulous, breathy, hurried manner of speaking that at times resembles a stutter; or slow, halting speech patterns peppered with inappropriate stops and repeating sounds
- A general lack of volume and force, the voice frequently dropping to an almost inaudible level
- Sudden pauses or long stops in the middle of a sentence made while attempting to recall a word or thought
- A monotonous and uninflected voice tone with an absence of the energy, rhythm, and emphasis common to normal speech

In many cases, PD patients afflicted with speech problems are well advised to consult a speech-language pathologist/therapist. Speech therapists first perform an evaluation of the patient's speaking abilities, then provide recommendations and, if necessary, a course of therapy in speech improvement that lasts from several visits to three or four months, depending on the seriousness of the condition. These sessions teach basic techniques of speech enhancement and provide methods of compensation for impairments that cannot be therapeutically improved. A number of strategies exist in both areas, many of which can be practiced at home. The section below will acquaint you with the procedures that many speech therapists stress, and will help you determine whether speech therapy is needed in your own situation.

Three Types of Speech Impairment

Speech therapy is concerned with three areas of impairment: (1) articulation, (2) phrasing, and (3) voice volume and amplification.

Articulation

PD people with speech impairments tend to slur and mumble their words. Addressing this common problem, a therapist may start by teaching patients to exaggerate their pronunciation, over-stressing every syllable, and making magnified movements of the mouth and lips as they do. Jane Goldberg, a speech language pathologist at Nyack Hospital in Nyack, New York, says:

> I teach my patients to pretend that they're on stage and that they have to pronounce each syllable separately and distinctly the way an actor would do. At first they're concerned that this technique will make them sound foolish. I tell them that overemphasizing words in this way seems strange to them but to the world it sounds just fine. Remember, I tell them, the extra efforts you make to pronounce each syllable compensate for your weakened articulation skills. These exaggerations will make up for any weakness you have and will end up raising you to what for others is a normal conversational level of speech.

A standard exercise requires that patients repeat certain phrases in a slow, even manner, emphasizing every syllable of every word. These exercises should be done on a regular basis if they are to pay off, preferably several times a day. The examples given below are typical phrases:

Lots of fun	Horse around
Cup of soup	Knife and fork
Jump for joy	Participation pays
Sing for your supper	Gang of boys
Chunk of cheese	Package of carrots
Vanilla flavoring	Stand back, Stuart
Make a phone call	Gretchen's garden

Patients pronounce each phrase as crisply as they can, taking pains to sound out the individual parts:

Lot-sss ah fa-nnn

Joh-mp forrrr jo-ee

Par-tiss-uh-pay-shun pay-zzz

Since there are many words in English that can be sounded out by ignoring the vowels and exaggerating the consonants, patients are drilled in sentences where the consonants transmit the full meaning. This is an interesting concept and one worth considering. For example, a phrase such as "Scotch tape" can be clearly communicated by stressing only the consonants and specifically the plosives (a word that requires closure of the oral passage such as "Scotch"). It's a trick, really, done by exaggerating the "skhah" sound in "Scotch," almost coughing it out from the back of the throat, then raising the upper lip and aggressively sounding out the "ch" sound. Result: "Skhah-ch!" The mouth itself does all the work. It is the same for "tape." Loudly "tsk" out the "tay" sound, then pop the "p": "tay-ph!" This phrase is manufactured entirely by the lips, tongue, and throat, with the voice playing a minimal part. Practice with other phrases:

Come quickly (Kmmmm! Kwwww-kah-leeeee!)

Sit here (Ssss-ttt! Hhhh-rrrrraaahhhh!)

Take it off (Tah-kkkkkhhh! Eeettttt! Ffffff!)

Fine kettle of fish

TV show

Chocolate cheesecake

Charley chucks chickens

Cupcake kid

When people articulate words they use four parts of their mouth in various combination to do the job: their lips, teeth, tongue, and throat. Articulation exercises are thus designed to work on all four parts.

One set of exercises, for instance, has patients repeating words that stress hard consonant sounds like "k" and "j" at the end of a word (PD people with speech impairments tend to drop their final consonants). These are sounded at the back of the throat. Try them: rake, wreck, peg, bag, bug, back, jig, jag, jug, lake, lock, lick, like, chunk. Repeat these words every day several times.

A second exercise uses words formed by touching the tongue either to the roof of the mouth or to the front of the teeth, especially the "d," "l," "n," "s," "t," and "sh" sounds such as touch, teeth, shout, lie, little, temple, sitting, tiptoe, shiny, neon, meaning, mighty, nod, nettle, necktie.

A third exercise stresses the "b," "f," "m," "p," and "v" sounds formed by the lips and teeth. Examples include pill, probe, phobic, bike, baseball, funny, fine, fiddle, pick, poke, pundit, very, volleyball, vice president, mica, merry, Mickey Mouse, mammal, memory, mimosa.

To give patients feedback in these exercises, they are encouraged to speak the words into a tape recorder, then to play back the results, listening carefully to each phrase and identifying specific areas where they are weak or unclear. Some therapists advise patients to look into a mirror while performing the exercises and to make corrections for faulty lip or mouth movements.

Participants are asked to practice these phrases at home for ten or twenty minutes a day. An excellent collection of such exercises is available in a pamphlet entitled "Speech Problems and Swallowing Problems in Parkinson's Disease" available from the American Parkinson Disease Association (call toll-free 800-223-APDA for ordering information).

Phrasing

A second area of concern for speech-impaired PD people is phrasing. Problems in this department are caused by weak motor control of the tongue and mouth muscles, both of which cause patients to talk in droning, uninflected, monotone sentences that speed up or slow down arrhythmically and which often become inaudible before they are complete. Word emphasis, stress, accent, rhythm—all the elements that make conversation lively and communicative are reduced.

To improve phrasing, therapists encourage patients to make minute pauses after each word, and to break up their words into individually pronounced syllables: I am go-ing to the su-per-market. The tem-per-a-ture is com-for-table to-day.

This maneuver is demanding, and patients often believe it sounds strange and artificial to other people. But again, if the exercise is done correctly it compensates for impaired speech patterns and makes sentences sound relatively normal. If the pauses are noticed at all by others, which they often are not, listeners simply assume that the patient is a slow talker and has something very worthwhile to say. Meanwhile, the patient is understood—and that's what it's all about.

For practice in word-by-word phrasing patients are encouraged to read out loud from a newspaper or book every day, purposefully pausing after every word or so, and making conscious efforts to pronounce sentences in measured, rhythmical beats. A tape recorder is again a handy resource for feedback. Speaking slowly is the key.

Voice Volume and Amplification

It is difficult to speak normally if one's breath is weak and projection is impaired. Though attitudes are divided among speech pathologists concerning how much help can actually be given to patients for this problem, a number of exercises do exist both to strengthen breath control and to teach compensation techniques for the lack of it.

CONTROLLED BREATHING.   Before beginning a session of exercise patients open their mouth halfway and breathe deeply eight or ten times, concentrating on taking a short breath in and exhaling a long breath out.

CONTROLLED PHONATION.   Patients breathe in, then out. On the out breath they intone the vowel sound "ah" for as long as possible. Fifteen to twenty seconds is a reasonable goal. They continue this same exercise with other vowel combinations, voicing a protracted "ay," "aw," "ee," "eye," "oh," "ow," "ouu," on each out breath. The same exercise is practiced using numbers instead of vowels, counting "one," "two," "three."

TAKING FREQUENT BREATHS.   The weakness of the respiratory muscles in PD and the consequent lack of amplification and duration make it advisable for patients to take a breath before beginning each new sentence. The longer the phrase that must be pronounced, the more necessary it is to breathe first. Some therapists encourage patients to break up each sentence with several breaths, or even to take a quick breath before each word. Try for a steady sound even if the duration is brief.

SUCCESSIVE AMPLIFICATION.   Patients begin by saying a sentence in their normal voice: "The cat jumped over the moon." They pause a moment, take a breath, then repeat the same sentence in a louder voice. They then pause again and repeat it in a *very* loud voice. Using similar three- or four-word sentences, they repeat each sentence three times, increasing voice volume each time.

INFLECTION EXERCISE.   Patients make up a simple declarative sentence such as: "I don't want another piece of cake." They repeat this sentence the first time emphasizing the first word: *"I* don't want another piece of cake." On the second repetition they emphasize the next word: I *don't* want another piece of cake." On the third: I don't *want* another piece of cake. And so on to the end of the sentence.

SINGING.   People are encouraged to sing favorite tunes at the top of their lungs, belting them out with as much volume and gusto as they can muster. The simple (and sometimes forgotten) pleasure of singing will be a spirit lifter and will often have a subtle improving influence on voice quality. As with many aspects of PD, motivation, emotion, and conscious effort play a large part in influencing one's symptoms. "Why is it," asks a spouse of a PD person, "that my husband mumbles so much of the time *except* when he's telling me off? Then he's as loud and clear as a bell!"

MECHANICAL VOICE AMPLIFIERS.   When projection and volume are a particular problem patients can purchase portable microphones that clip onto the vest pocket or rest on the table. Be aware, however, that these devices are in the developmental stage and that they are far from a cure-all for voice volume difficulties. Moreover, if slurring and poor phrasing are a problem along with projection, the amplifier will do nothing more than increase these impairments. ("If your radio is full of static," says speech language pathologist Jane Goldberg, "you don't turn up the volume.") At the same time, many patients consider amplifiers to be a real help. Consult with a doctor or with a speech pathologist on this one.

Amplifiers are made by Radio Shack (try your local branch), Bell Telephone Company (talk to your local Bell office), Park Surgical Company (5001 New Utrecht Avenue, Brooklyn, NY 11219; 718-436-9200), and the Luminaud Company (8680 Tyler Blvd., Mentor, OH 44060; 216-255-9082). They sell for around two hundred dollars and up.

Facial Mobility Exercises

A number of facial exercises are now used for PD people to help loosen up the muscles of the mouth, tongue, and jaw before speaking. These exercises help both with speaking and with improving lack of facial expression. Exercises you can do at home include:

• Open your mouth wide for several moments. Then close it so that your lips are tightly sealed. Repeat several times.

• Pucker your mouth and blow through your lips with a steady breath. Repeat three or four times. Whistle for several minutes.

• Suck your cheeks in, hold, then relax. Repeat several times. Puff your cheeks out, hold, then relax. Repeat several times.

- Scrunch up your face. Repeat several times. Make an exaggerated smile, then an exaggerated frown. Repeat several times.

- Wrinkle your nose. Move your eyebrows up and down. Knit your brow. Wiggle your ears and scalp. Tighten and release your Adam's apple. Jut your chin out and back. Extend your lower lip. Smack your lips and pucker them.

- Stick your tongue out as far as it will go. Move your tongue around in circles. Try to touch your nose with your tongue. Lick your lips in a circular motion. Stick your tongue out to the right side of your mouth, then to the left. Alternate several times. Dart your tongue in and out like a snake. Curl your tongue and touch it to the back of your throat.

Note: All of the above exercises can be practiced with a tongue depressor to increase resistance and to give the tongue a better workout. When done a few minutes before dinner, these exercises will facilitate chewing and swallowing.

For the Caregiver

Caregivers often tend to finish sentences for patients or to speak in their place. Be careful of this. Let patients do their own talking.

Encourage patients to speak slowly and, if necessary, to rephrase incoherent sentences into simpler and more direct language. A weighty idea can usually be reduced from one long, meandering sentence to several short, simple ones. Also, keep emphasizing to the patient the importance of body language and of gesture and expression. A shake of the head or a raise of an eyebrow is often all that needs to be "said" on the subject. Remember, communication is the goal. Whether it be verbal or nonverbal doesn't matter much.

If you want to encourage a patient to speak slowly, provide a role model: Speak in loud, measured, paced tones yourself, and encourage patients to do the same. After a while slow speech will become a habit for both of you.

When communicating with patients, encourage them to

speak in complete sentences rather than to nod or grunt or give a yes-no answer. Properly phrased questions will help. For instance, instead of asking "Do you want some tea?" which can be answered with a shake of the head, say "I'll get you some tea. What kind do you want? Do you want cream or sugar in it?" Or instead of "Do you want to wear your blue jacket?" try "What jacket would you like to wear today?" Led on by this tactic, patients gain speaking practice while communication between parties is improved.

Be aware, finally, that though the patient may work closely with a speech therapist and may develop a number of sophisticated compensatory communication strategies, these methods. are difficult to implement and tiring to sustain. Therapists often recommend that at home, in the security and noncompetitive atmosphere of the household, the patient should be allowed to slur, speak softly, and even to drool. There will be opportunity enough for patients to make communication efforts in the outside world.

Further Hints for Improving Speech

• Before you begin to speak, swallow first. This will clear your mouth of saliva and prevent drooling and/or choking.

• Be aware of atmospheric and ambient noise. Talking when the TV is on or when children are crying is a sure way to mar a conversation. Physical positioning is important too. For example, to enhance body language and directness of interaction always face the person with whom you are speaking. At a table in a restaurant, position yourself so that you can be heard easily by the waiter and by other people.

• If a PD patient has insufficient voice volume to call out from room to room, use a household intercom. This is an especially useful resource in a two-story house or in homes where one person spends most of the time, say, in the kitchen and the other in the bedroom or den.

• When in public make a conscious effort to speak more loudly than usual. This added 20 percent volume may be just what's needed to bring your voice up to normal conversational level.

• Speaker telephones or phone voice amplifiers are a must for people with volume difficulties. They are available from most appliance or radio and TV stores.

• Encourage patients with severe voice impairment to carry a pad and pen with them, and to write down all important messages.

NOTES

1. With thanks for this tip to J. David Grimes, M.D., Peggy Gray, R.N., and Kelly Grimes, B.Sc., in their very useful book *Parkinson's Disease . . . One Step at a Time* published by the Parkinson's Society of Ottawa-Carleton, 1989, 51.
2. J. Rozovski and S. Laurie, *Nutrition and Parkinson's Disease, Some Information and Recommendations* (Columbia University Medical Center, New York: Parkinson's Disease Foundation).
3. Roger C. Duvoisin, M.D., *Parkinson's Disease: A Guide for Patient and Family* (New York: Raven Press, 1984), 131–132.

14

Resources, Advice, and Equipment That Really Help

For Parkinson's sufferers, pulling a shirt over the head or bending down to tie a shoe can become a struggle fraught with risks, an encounter with gravity, equilibrium, and a hard floor that looms a long, long way down. The same is true for walking to the bathroom at night; or threading a needle, striking a match, climbing in and out of a shower stall, slicing a tomato—these and a thousand other seemingly simple activities of daily living loom large on the horizon of many PD people, no longer automatic chores but formidable hurdles which must be approached with concentrated caution and sometimes even dread. For PD people, nothing that concerns the activities of daily living can ever be taken for granted.

Occupational therapists, health-care professionals, and medical equipment manufacturers have all brought the full focus of their ingenuity to bear on the daily living problems faced by PD people, and today there are many aids and resources, both physical and informational, that make the life of mobility-restricted people easier and less complex than ever before. This chapter, based on recent aid product developments for the movement-impaired and on interviews with doctors and occupational therapists, profiles these resources.

Especially to be stressed are the many useful and ingenious articles of orthopedic and ADL (activities of daily living) equipment designed for mobility-restricted people. Finally, note that when specific orthopedic items are mentioned in the paragraphs that follow, the source for each will be given in parentheses. The complete names and addresses of these companies will then be provided in full at the end of the chapter. (With special thanks for information provided here by Barbara Berry, OTR and supervising occupational therapist at Nyack Hospital.)

GETTING DRESSED AND UNDRESSED

Depending on how much rigidity and slowness one suffers from, dressing in the morning and undressing at night can be problematic, with the main difficulties centering on stiffness, loss of balance, and lack of manual dexterity. There is help for all three.

To begin, many occupational therapists recommend that patients remain seated while dressing and undressing in order to reduce all possibilities of falling. For those who regularly find themselves doing battle with buttons, Velcro tabs make excellent replacements. Attaching a ring or tab pull to a zipper will make zipping an easier chore. Note, by the way, that though many health-care suppliers offer a variety of mechanical "buttoners" that are reputed to make buttoning and unbuttoning trouble-free, the general consensus among PD people interviewed is that they cause more problems than they cure.

As far as footwear goes, many stores offer a line of shoes that feature snaps or Velcro closures in place of laces. Loafers make good alternatives too. Long-handled shoe horns are a valuable aid for people who have difficulty bending at the waist (Cleo). One model, the hemiplegia shoe horn, holds the shoe in place and makes foot insertion more efficient (Cleo). People who require help putting on socks will find stocking pull-on devices available from several sources (Sammons, Cleo, Mature Wisdom).

For women, reaching behind to fasten a bra is hard on both the arms and the shoulder joints. Front closure bras with modified camisole elastic straps will eliminate this problem entirely (Enrichments). Sweaters that button or snap down the front go on more easily than the pullover variety. The same is true for shirts or dresses. Slip-over nightgowns, on the other hand, generally require less of a struggle than pajamas.

People who have trouble with belt fasteners are advised to trade in their buckling models for the snap, slip-in, or Velcro varieties. Pants with built-in waist elastic such as sweat pants will eliminate this inconvenience completely. (Men find suspenders a help too.)

An all-purpose dressing aid that many patients swear by is the dressing stick, a multipurpose hooked prod that pulls up socks, hitches pants, yanks zippers, reaches across the bed or onto high hooks for dresses—you name it (Arthritis Self-Help Products).

SAFETY IN THE BATHROOM

Statistically speaking, falls in wet tubs or bathroom floors account for more accidents to Parkinson's patients than any other domestic mishap. Grab bars and safety rails are the number one priority here and are well worth the price of purchase and installation. Bars and rails come in all colors and lengths, some plastic coated, some stainless steel, many in coordinated colors and decorator finish. Catalog photos will help you decide which model best suits your decor (Cleo, Sammons, Enrichments, Mature Wisdom).

Another pragmatic piece of apparatus is the raised toilet seat, a portable molded plastic seat that increases the height of the toilet bowl from 2 to 6 inches and fits over any standard-size porcelain bowl. This ingenious piece of equipment is a real boon for those who find regular-size seats too low for comfort, or who encounter difficulty when they try to stand after using the facilities. It comes in all shapes and sizes including adjustable and cushioned seats, seats with built-in arms, and portable traveling models (Cleo, Sammons, Enrichments). A related aid is the adjustable toilet safety rail that serves as an armrest and a push-off support (Enrichments, Cleo, Sammons).

For bathing, many physical and occupational therapists recommend bathtub seats. These handy supports come in a variety of models, both the four-legged stool kind that sits in the middle of the tub, and the flat, across-the-top variety that adjusts to fit bathtub width. The value of such seats is twofold: They encourage bathers to sit rather than stand while showering, reducing the risk of falls, and they provide better seating for those who find it difficult to lower themselves into the bottom of a tub (Cleo, Sammons, Enrichments).

An intriguing variation on the basic tub stool is the Bathomatic Hydrocushion, a water-inflatable seat that can be filled from the tap until it expands into a cushy pillow seat that is both stable and, if need be, portable (Enrichments). Those who prefer to stand while showering will want to lay down a toe-grip bath mat plus textured safety treads (Enrichments).

If your bathroom floor is especially hard and if you've lost a drinking glass or two to it already, use paper cups instead of glass. For men, if your tremor is unpredictable, an electric shaver will help avoid nicks and cuts. Similarly, an electric toothbrush is easier to manipulate than a manual model. Another useful item is the Little Octopus, a suction cup that holds soap to the shower wall or drinking glasses to the sink basin (Cleo).

Other useful washing and toilet aids include long-handled sponges, soapers, and scrub brushes (Mature Wisdom, Enrichments, Cleo, Arthritis Self-Help Products); soap on a rope (the drugstore); inflatable back pillows for lying comfortably in a bathtub (Enrichments, Cleo); hand-held shower heads for seated showering (Enrichments); portable tub grab bars to use when traveling (Enrichments); curved bath brushes for easy access to the back, neck, and shoulder regions (Cleo); soaper mit for washing with one hand (Cleo); and male and female urinals to eliminate stumbling nighttime walks to the bathroom (Cleo).

GROOMING AIDS

If you have trouble positioning yourself in front of the bathroom or bedroom mirror, let the mirror come to you: extension mirrors attach to a folding accordion spring and can be set at any angle or distance you choose (Cleo). Another model, the Flex-A-Mirror, is mounted on a long, flexible shaft and is bent to any position desired (Cleo).

People with unsteady hands may wish to trim their nails with a toe clipper rather than conventional nail cutters—it's easier. A nail brush and cloth nail file with suction cups on the bottom are also useful (Cleo).

People with especially stiff joints may wish to avail themselves of adjustable combs and brushes. Mounted on long handles, these handy tools adjust to whatever angle is desired and lock in place for easy grooming (Enrichments, Sammons). A full line of easy-grip orthopedic brushes is also available (Cleo).

EATING

For people whose tremor causes liquid spills at mealtime, the humble flexible straw will help. Plastic glasses with extra wide bases likewise prevent accidents (Cleo).

For those with neck rigidity, a glass with a special notch cut to fit the nose allows eaters to drink without leaning their heads back or craning their necks forward (Cleo). Special plates with raised rims and stick-to-the-bottom surfaces permit people with impaired manual dexterity to eat comfortably with one hand (Cleo, Enrichments).

In the silverware department, large-handled knives, spoons, and forks ensure a firm grip; so do weighted or foam-padded utensils (Cleo, Enrichments) and the one-handed roller knife and curved handle spoon (Cleo). Another interesting tool that eliminates the need for constantly changing from one utensil to another is the "spork," a combination steel spoon and fork (Cleo). Other orthopedically designed plates, cups, and eating instruments are available from all the sources listed at the end of this chapter.

MAKING KITCHEN WORK EASIER

A remarkable array of kitchen aids for the movement-impaired has been developed over the past twenty years, and here we can profile only a few of the most useful and interesting items. A typical selection includes:

• One-handed rolling pin, can opener, and eggbeater for people with limited manual dexterity (Enrichments, Sammons).

• All-purpose bottle and jar openers. These come in a number of models and varieties (Enrichments, Cleo, Sammons, Arthritis Self-Help Products).

• Nonslip graters and slicers. Both pieces of equipment stay put on the counter due to nonslip suction bases (Enrichments).

• Stay-put twin suction disks for temporarily attaching one flat surface to another, for example, a mixing bowl to a counter top (Cleo).

• Stainless steel bowl and bowl holder. A plated metal frame holds a bowl firmly in place while the mixing is done (Sammons).

• Stay-put cutting board with suction cups on the bottom and a clamp on the side to keep things steady (Cleo).

• Nonslip surface material. Two-sided pieces will hold dishes, bowls, plates, and so forth in place (Cleo).

• One-handed electric can opener. A freestanding model designed especially for one-handed or limited-range-of-motion operation (Cleo).

• Grocery grip. A padded handle with hook designed to carry one or several bags at a time (Arthritis Self-Help Products).

• Stove valve turner. A triangular grip fits various sizes and types of stoves and makes knob turning easier (Cleo). Of similar use is the Uni-Turner from Enrichments.

• No-hands refrigerator door opener. Just step on a floor lever and open (Enrichments).

• Revolving tray. Keep one in the refrigerator and/or on the dining table at all times. It makes reaching easier for everyone (available at any hardware or house goods store).

• Kettle tilter is adjustable to fit any kettle from 6.25 to 8 inches in diameter. It eliminates lifting and is perfect for PD people with weak wrists (Cleo).

HELP WITH HOUSEWORK

Household chores can be accomplished more efficiently with help from both common sense and modern therapeutic ingenuity. For example, if bending over to vacuum is a problem, long-handled carpet sweepers will do the job almost as well and they demand far fewer back contortions. A long-handled dust pan and broom, available at most hardware stores, accomplishes the same task. If you must reach up to dust, dusters can be mounted on long poles. Long-handled dusters can also be purchased (Enrichments).

If you frequently move tables and chairs around your house put casters on commonly moved items. A wheeled table known as the Versatilt changes height and angle, and supports up to 50 pounds of household items (Enrichments, Arthritis Self-Help Products).

Housework demands the constant use of spray cans, and here a slip-on handle known as the Push Button Pusher makes it easier to depress caps (Enrichments). For one-handed scrubbing the suction scrub brush adheres to counters or sinks (Enrichments).

Perhaps the handiest of all household aids is the automatic extension arm, a long, lightweight plastic or aluminium pole with a lock grip attached to one end. Just reach for the wanted item, depress the trigger at the base of the pole, and the gripper does the rest. Some models include a magnet on the gripper for lifting metallic objects. This one is employable for a thousand jobs and comes recommended by many PD people (Arthritis Self-Help Products, Cleo, Sammons).

IN BED

Sheets made of silk, satin, or any sleek materials will give more slide and will make it easier to roll over in bed. Nightgowns or pajamas composed of similar materials help in the same way. A truly valuable bedside aid is the helping handle, a portable, attachable vinyl-coated steel grip that clamps onto any standard-size bed and provides hand support for sitting up or rolling over. Take it with you when you travel (Arthritis Self-Help Products).

PD people are frequently sensitive to the weight of heavy blankets. A frame blanket support eliminates this problem, allowing freedom of leg movement while providing ample warmth for the feet (Mature Wisdom). If lower back and hip rigidity causes pain, a wedge-shaped contoured cushion elevates the legs and takes pressure off the lower back (Mature Wisdom, Arthritis Self-Help Products).

A number of interesting orthopedic pillows are now available, one of the most popular being the variable density pillow that features a soft section at one end, a hard section at the other, and medium density in the middle (Arthritis Self-Help Products, Mature Wisdom). Another popular model, the Ortho pillow, is shaped like an hourglass and is specifically designed for people with a stiff and chronically sore neck (Arthritis Self-Help Products).

Finally, if fine-tuning the knobs and levers of an alarm clock is an irritation, the Talking Alarm Clock can be set with the push of a single button and will gently wake you up with a rooster-like crow (Mature Wisdom). Another talking model, the Spartus Talking Alarm, features volume control, auto voice, and hourly time announcements (Products for People with Vision Problems).

AT THE DESK

If regular scissors no longer do the job, a line of orthopedic models are available from several manufacturers (Enrichments, Arthritis Self-Help Products). Reading stands, sold at any hardware or stationery store, are helpful for arranging books and papers at the right viewing angle and for making page turning easier. Automatic page turners are also available (Cleo).

Pens and pencils for the writing-impaired come in a wide and perhaps bewildering variety. Most are designed to solve two basic problems: poor grip and lack of pressure on the point. For starters, there are precut, slip-on pen and pencil grips. These plastic tubes and triangles slide onto most writing instruments and greatly improve their gripability (Arthritis Self-Help Products). (Multicolored models can be purchased from Enrichments.) A plastic pen holder that straps on the back of the hand is another alternative (Cleo), as is the weighted ballpoint pen that provides pen-point pressure from the weight of the instrument alone, and works for even the weakest hand (Cleo). The Wanchik writer supports the hand and keeps the pen or pencil automatically aligned (Enrichments).

There's the Arthwriter, a lightweight, easily gripped plastic ball with a hole in the center to hold pen or pencil (Cleo). The Rheumatics Pen, shaped with a special thumb-fold grip, is designed for those with impaired hand and arm movements (Cleo). The biocurve pen is engineered to take pressure off the fingers and wrist, and is excellent for people with wrist joint rigidity (Arthritis Self-Help Products). Finally, if the choice between all these writing instruments is overwhelming, you can simply use a felt-tip pen. This ubiquitous writing instrument requires little or no pressure on the point and produces a quality of line second to none.

COMMUNICATIONS

Perhaps the greatest boon modern communications has bestowed on the PD patient is the cordless telephone. This item is not cheap, but it does save the annoyance of leaping up each time the phone rings, racing from room to room, climbing stairs, tripping over cords, and so on. Models are available at any appliance or radio and TV store. Speaker phones are handy for people who have trouble gripping receivers, though beware of the cheaper models: They tend to malfunction after several months of use.

Telephones with one-button dialing are a pragmatic asset for people who have diminished fine motor movements of the fingers. Another boon along these lines is a set of large push buttons that fit over the ordinary buttons on most phones (Enrichments). For those who are seeing-impaired, large-print dials are a practical aid (Products for People with Vision Problems). Another resource along the same lines is the large-number dual-power calculator that has 1-inch-high numbers programmed into the display window (Mature Wisdom).

MAKING THINGS SAFE AROUND THE HOUSE

If balance loss is a recurring worry take up all scatter rugs. At the minimum, make sure they are firmly tacked or taped to the floor. Be wary of frayed or ragged rug ends that catch the feet. In general, carpeting is a better alternative for floor covering than loose rugs: It cuts noise, improves traction, and softens impact in case of falls. If any sharp cornered furniture is in the line of a possible fall, move it, or at least cover its exposed edges.

If you awaken frequently at night, install night lights in your bedroom, bathroom, kitchen, stairways, and hallways for midnight meandering. Grab bars installed in much used rooms—not necessarily just the bathroom—may save you a fall.

Keep several flashlights and a box of candles handy in different parts of the home in case of a blackout or emergency. If you frequently move small objects from room to room, a portable wheeled cart (such as a grocery cart) will make the job easier.

Be sure your staircase areas are safe. Remember that all uncarpeted or uncovered stairs are slippery stairs, especially if the nosing on the edge of the tread is rounded. Nonslip tape, rubber treads, or strip carpeting will reduce these hazards severalfold. Just be sure all stair coverings are meticulously tacked down. Loose rugs make staircases a danger zone.

All staircases should likewise have a securely mounted banister, with nonskid tape secured to its underside to increase grip security. Keep the lighting in this area as bright as possible; lights are a must here (a light that turns on automatically as night comes is available from Arthritis Self-Help Products). If a fall does occur on the stairs, it will cause a good deal less harm if pointed objects (such as tables, chairs, umbrella stands) have previously been removed from the bottom of the landing—some people arrange extra padding at the foot of the stairs as well.

Make sure that all walkways leading up to your home are evenly graded, and that jutting roots, broken cobblestones, and uneven gravel surfaces are eliminated. If front door steps turn slippery after inclement weather, their treads can be covered with rubber runners. These sometimes come in different colors, a boon for visibility to everyone.

For improved seating comfort, add several cushions or seat supports to sofas and chairs. These raise the level of a person's knees and back, and make it easier to get in and out of chairs. Leg base extenders that raise the height of chair seats from 3 to 6 inches serve the same purpose (Enrichments, Sammons).

Other aids for ease of living include snap-on knob extensions for easier gripping (Enrichments, Cleo), plastic car door openers (Cleo, Enrichments), light switch extension handles (Cleo), leverage key turners (Enrichments), and lamp turn-on extension levers (Sammons).

The names and addresses of health supplies featured in this chapter are as follows:

Arthritis Self-Help Products
3 Little Knoll Ct.
Medford, NJ 08055
609-654-6918

Cleo, Inc.
3957 Mayfield Rd.
Cleveland, OH 44121
800-321-0595

Enrichments for Better Living
145 Tower Dr.
P.O. Box 579
Hinsdale, IL 60521
800-323-5547

Mature Wisdom
Hanover, PA 17333-0028
800-638-6366

Products for People with Vision Problems
Consumer Products
American Federation for the Blind
15 W. 16th St.
New York, NY 10011
212-862-8838

Sammons, Inc.
Box 32
Brookfield, IL 60513-0032
800-323-5547
(Orders from Sammons must be made through a health-care
professional.)

15

Getting Help from Others: A Patient and Caregiver's Guide

Sometimes the patient and/or the caregiver simply cannot go it alone. Support of some kind is needed. Perhaps loneliness sets in with a vengeance. The patient is bored sitting home all day with nothing to do but mope over his or her situation. Or the caregiver is tired of never getting a break from the same old routine. Perhaps physical or occupational therapy of some kind is required; or psychological counseling; or an exercise program, religious guidance, or just a friendly pat on the shoulder and a sympathetic smile. The type of assistance required by each person will be different. But be assured that somewhere along the line, at some time, outside help will be a welcome option.

And help is available from more sources than you might think. Indeed, if you live in an American city of even moderate size, most of the resources listed in this chapter will be available to you in one form or another. More effort will be necessary to gain access in rural areas, of course, though as Parkinson's disease continues to increase among the general population, support groups and agencies of all kinds are popping up everywhere. In general, if you need help it will be there. The most important thing is that you seek it. Here's how.

IF YOU LIVE ALONE

Patients who live by themselves or who spend a majority of time alone while family members are in the workplace require special assistance, both to help maintain an active social life and to make certain that enough safety factors are available to ensure peace of mind.

Start by making a point of getting out of your house at least once a day for at least an hour or two at a stretch—shopping, chatting with a friend, attending a social club, walking in the park. Force yourself if you have to.

If you are a homebound PD person you can still reach out to others via the telephone. Patients who belong to support groups make a point of phoning each other regularly. Receiving four or five calls daily from friends and fellow parkinsonians can break up the long hours. It can assure people that they count, and that they are still part of things.

Keep all important telephone numbers posted by your phone. These include numbers for family members, friends, the hospital, an ambulance service, the police, your local pharmacy, and all important medical professionals. Remember also to stock your medicine cabinet with a good first aid kit in case of falls or accidents. Make sure that family members and/or friends understand what to do in case of an emergency. Be sure they have all the necessary medical phone numbers and drug information on hand, and that they know how to perform CPR (cardiopulmonary resuscitation) and the Heimlich maneuver.

In case of an accident or unconsciousness, it is wise to carry a card in your wallet or purse describing your condition, listing the medicines you are taking, giving the names of your doctor and next of kin, and providing all appropriate medical directions and information.

If you drive, apply to the Department of Motor Vehicles for

a handicapped driver permit. This useful card allows you to park in easy-access areas, and in some states it exempts you from paying parking meter fees.

Another helpful safety aid is telephone reassurance service. This is an organized volunteer program whose members call one another at designated hours of the day or night. If patients do not answer the phone at the scheduled call times, or if something is wrong when they do, the caller goes to the person's home and/or gets in touch with a physician. You can even organize your own telephone reassurance service with the help of a booklet on the subject from the Administration on Aging. Write for catalog: OHD 75-20200, USGPO, Washington, D.C.

A rather expensive but potentially lifesaving resource for PD people who live alone is a phone-care electronic hookup that is tied into a central location like the police station or a private monitoring agency. Installed directly in the patient's house, one version of this device sends out a beeping sound at regular intervals; if the signal is not switched off at a designated hour the alarm automatically triggers a prerecorded emergency call to several people including the patient's doctor, family members, or friends. A medical professional or hospital referral service will be able to tell you about programs available in your area.

FINDING GOOD COUNSELING

At times, PD people simply need to talk. There are several options.

Psychologists and Psychiatrists

In some cases, the strain of living with PD or of having a spouse with the disease becomes so intense that one's self-managing skills begin to fail and long-term psychological help is required. How can you tell when this moment has arrived? Is there an ultimate sign patients or caregivers can look for that signals the need for professional aid? Yes, there is. It is simple: If you feel you can no longer cope, then you can't.

The need for professional assistance is a subjective matter that depends to a large extent on a person's own perceptions: If you *think* you need help, you do. Period. Every person has their own threshold, of course, and everyone must decide for themselves when the time has come. For one person a depression that won't quit is the straw that breaks the camel's back. For another it is an obsessive eating binge, a series of panic attacks, suicidal ideations, dependence on alcohol or sedatives, or a habitual feeling of being out of control. Whatever one's psychological fuse point may be, know that each of us *does* have this point, and that to go beyond it without asking for help is to endanger your deepest emotional well-being.

Referrals for mental health assistance are usually made through a physician. Support groups can also advise, as can other PD patients. Positive word of mouth from satisfied clients is the best of all recommendations in this department.

Social Workers

Over the past decade more and more social workers have gone into counseling practice. Trained to deal with both crisis intervention and a client's practical medical and social needs, social workers are often the ideal professionals to turn to for acute, short-term problems such as family disputes, coping with a recent medical diagnosis, grief therapy, discharge planning, and medical referrals.

Usually less expensive than psychologists and psychiatrists, social workers can be a perfect alternative for those who feel they need counseling with practical concerns of daily living as well as with social and emotional problems.

Religious Counseling

Sometimes questions that arise in the minds of PD patients and their caregivers are questions not so much of body as of soul: "Why am I sick?" "Why must I suffer?" "Why will I die?" When such thoughts begin to take up more and more of the day, many PD people find that their greatest comfort comes not from friends and not from close family but from a religious group.

We live in a time when many people have forgotten that the religious alternative exists. One rarely finds it mentioned in the endless number of books written today on becoming self-fulfilled and anxiety-free. Yet, religious counseling and contemplation are there, calling to those so inclined. Clerics of all persuasions are available for those who feel the need.

Physical and Occupational Therapists

In the chapter on exercise we have seen how large a part physical therapists can play in helping PD people live a healthy, happy life. These highly trained professionals are major allies for PD people and can start them on exercise and physical self-help programs that will become a major part of the overall therapy plan.

Likewise, occupational therapists are trained to enter a person's home, make a complete evaluation, and help patients design their lives so that the activities of daily living become more manageable. Members of both these professions can be hired for in-home consultation from a health-care agency, or they can be consulted directly at local hospitals.

Support Groups

Of all the social, emotional, and moral boosts a PD person can get, many patients agree that nothing surpasses membership in a Parkinson's support group. Whereas friends may look away and stammer their excuses, whereas associates may think they understand your dilemma but don't, whereas the world may minimize or even ignore the struggle you are engaged in every day, members of a support group are different. They have been there. They know things firsthand. They can help.

Janet C.: I go for companionship and to meet people who are in the same boat as myself. They're the only ones who really understand what having Parkinson's is all about. The doctors don't really.

Dave De R.: I have gotten *so* many good tips from other people at these meetings. These people have really thought things out, and remember, some have had Parkinson's for ten or fifteen years—that's a lot of time and experience to pass on to others.

Mary P.: My local group is the best. I've been to several but I like this one the most because the people there get so close to each other. Family, kind of. You become very close to people who share your fears and your hopes. People are open there in a way they're not elsewhere.

Mary G.: It's better here than out in the world. It's like going to a protected haven for an hour each week. We do a lot of things together too after the meetings, like group picnics and socializing. Going out to dinner. Calling each other. It's fun.

Ralph Z.: My dyskinesia gets so bad that I'm embarrassed to go out into public at times. At the Parkinson's group I don't get embarrassed at all. They understand there. The shaking and all my carrying on doesn't bother anyone.

Pearl B.: I get lonely and so I go to the group for friendship. People are nice to me there.

Sadler V.: I learn a lot. Some of these persons, I swear, know more about Parkinson's disease than the doctors. Maybe if the doctors had it for a couple of weeks they might pay more attention to the concerns that get talked about in the group like what to eat, vitamin E, ways of getting around, driving a car. How to get in and out of a car. How to get up from a park bench when your back hurts. What medications go with each other. How to cut a pill in half when you're shaking so bad you can hardly hold the razor. Things that help you get along. I learn tricks from the people at my group about living every time I go.

When like-minded people gather to talk and to help each other something good takes place. Information gets transmitted and people learn things they never knew before. But more subtly, emotions are exchanged; messages of the heart are passed around that sometimes change a person's life and give one hope to go on. Nothing else we know of—no therapy, no medication, no orthopedic aid, no exercise program—accomplishes this job quite as well. It comes only when people talk to people in a room full of trust and concern.

What gets discussed at a PD group? Anything that members wish to talk about, really. Typical subjects might include any of the following:

When and how to best take medications
Dealing with side effects
Depression and stress
Sleep problems
Ways to sit and stand up
New drugs and future technologies
Caregiving hints
Nursing skills
Dealing with lawyers and estate planning
Writing wills
Finding the best price for health care and medicines
Hobbies
Ins and outs of health insurance, Medicare, Medicaid, Social
    Security
Home safety
Nursing homes

The best doctors
Dealing with social embarrassment
Balance and falling

In some groups, caregivers and patients split into separate groups to discuss concerns specific to their needs and interest. In others, a caregiver's meeting will be held one week, a patient's meeting the next. A certain period of time is usually set aside in most groups for exercise, speech therapy, guest speakers, and socializing. Dues are always minimal.

You will find meetings of PD support groups held in hospitals, town halls, churches, schools, senior centers, or municipal buildings. Wherever they are, they help. Even if you don't think of yourself as a joiner, consider giving them a try. The chances are good that you will be pleasantly surprised.

Where do you find a PD group? Ask your doctor, a healthcare professional, or the information desk at your local hospital. Another alternative is to get in touch with one of the national Parkinson's organizations for referrals to local groups. The most prominent of these are mentioned below. Note that the American Parkinson Disease Association and the Parkinson's Educational Foundation both sponsor PD groups of their own across the country. You might also consider writing to these organizations for helpful booklets on PD, product and event information, and their very informative newsletters:

American Parkinson Disease Association
60 Bay St.
Staten Island, NY 10301

Parkinson's Disease Foundation
William Black Medical Research Building
Columbia Presbyterian Medical Center
New York, NY 10032

United Parkinson Foundation
360 W. Superior St.
Chicago, IL 60610

Parkinson's Educational Program
1800 Park Newport #302
Newport Beach, CA 92660

National Parkinson Foundation, Inc.
1501 Ninth Ave., N.W.
Miami, FL 33136

Parkinson's Disease Information and Referral Center
660 S. Euclid
Box 8111
St. Louis, MO 63110

Parkinson's Disease Foundation of Canada
Manulife Centre, Suite 232
55 Bloor St. W.
Toronto, Ontario M4W 1A6

Parkinson Foundation of Canada
Bureau 911
1155 Ave. Metculfe
Montreal, Quebec H3B 209

The Parkinson's Disease Society of the United Kingdom
36 Portland Pl.
London W1N 3DG, England

GETTING IN-HOME PROFESSIONAL HELP

Eventually the time may come when in-home professional nursing care becomes a necessity. This is especially likely if the PD patient lives alone or if the patient's spouse and/or family members are absent a majority of the day. The PD person may be immobilized and the caregiver may not be up to providing round-the-clock care. Some of the better options are discussed below.

Visiting Nurse Services

When a patient becomes wheelchair-bound, bed-bound, or extremely motion-impaired, in-home nursing services become the order of the day. In some instances, health insurance covers the rather extensive costs of these visits. Check your policy or talk to your insurance broker for details. In other cases, Medicare will help defray the bills, though a number of qualifications must be met first. Ask for the details from the Social Security Department that administers Medicare through the Health-Care Financing Administration.

There are, as a rule, two types of nurses available from home nursing services: licensed practical nurses and registered nurses. *Practical nurses* are graduates of a college nursing program or an accredited vocational school. They must pass a state board examination as well. Their skills are broad, qualifying them to perform a range of nursing services such as giving medications, washing and caring for the patient, maintaining a safe and comfortable household environment, and preparing a home-care plan.

Registered nurses are graduates of accredited colleges who have passed the state board examination and are licensed to practice with a physician and/or as independent agents. In general, registered nurses possess more skills and a wider range of medical knowledge than licensed nurses. They are also more expensive.

For information on visiting nurse services in your area speak with your physician, social worker, or with a discharge planner at a local hospital. You can also consult the yellow pages, though it's generally better to receive a personal referral first. Or you can get in touch directly with the following organizations for more information:

American Affiliation of Visiting Nurses
Associations and Services
21 Maryland Plaza
Suite 300
St. Louis, MO 63108

American Federation of Home Care
429 N Street S.W.
Suite S-605
Washington, DC 20024

Home Health Aids

One step down from accredited nurses in both skill and cost are home health aids. These men and women have usually received basic training in patient care, though not always a great deal. However, if all you need is someone in your home who knows how to make a bed and shop for groceries, a health aid is just what the doctor ordered.

What do home health aids do? As a rule they are trained to oversee personal-care chores such as bathing and toileting. They are experts at transport, able to move patients from one location to another in several different ways, and in dressing, feeding, and performing simple nursing chores such as taking vital signs, helping with exercise, and assisting with medication. In some instances, aids will provide domestic services such as light house-cleaning and cooking. Health aids can be hired through home-care agencies or via referrals from a medical professional.

In–Home Companions

Still another notch down in skill and price are in-home companions. They are usually untrained or semiskilled men and women who live with the patient full- or part-time, and who provide basic domestic services such as shopping, cooking, answering the phone, and cleaning. They also bring life and company to the house, and as such are often taken on simply as conversation mates and friends. In-home companions can be hired through a health-care agency or via referrals.

Homemakers

In many instances, a PD patient requires help with housework and general domestic duties. When needs arise, homemakers can be hired several days a week to help out at whatever tasks are called for: cleaning, taking out garbage, trimming hedges, lifting, carrying, whatever. Homemakers are hired directly from health-care agencies.

Other Home-Care Aids

Other helpers that PD patients may need at one time or another include nutritionists, speech therapists, chauffeur services, escort services, and chore workers. All can be provided by health-care agencies or via referrals.

Choosing a Home-Care Agency

Most large home health-care agencies provide all or at least a majority of the health-care services just listed. How can you tell the best agencies? Though there are no foolproof methods, here is a list of the questions you should ask before making your decision:

• How long has the agency been in business? Does it maintain several offices? Is it independent or part of a chain?

• How is the billing handled? Is the agency covered by insurance plans and Medicaid? Is it bonded (that is, if one of their employees steals from your home you receive reimbursement)? Does the agency maintain a sliding scale or part-pay program based on the client's income? Are there any hidden costs in billings such as transportation fees for workers? Can you get an itemized list of the services the agency provides *before* committing yourself?

• Does the agency offer a contract or service agreement stipulating its rates, services, specialists provided, hidden costs, and hours of care? What type of emergency response system does it offer?

• Is the agency certified or accredited? If not, why? Is it for profit or is it nonprofit? Can it provide references from doctors, administrators, community organizations, and hospitals? If not, why? Ask for specific names, and call these people directly.

• What type of training do the agency's in-home personnel receive? Ask for references.

• Does the agency provide home medical equipment? What kinds? What equipment is it *not* capable of providing? How does the billing work for equipment rentals?

• During what hours of the day and night does the agency provide services? Are services available on weekends? Holidays? Are fees higher for services provided during off hours? How much higher? Must you pay for a minimum number of hours even if you don't use them?

LEARNING MORE ABOUT PARKINSON'S DISEASE

Finally, one of the best ways to help yourself or the PD person is to know your subject. Knowledge is power, and it is available through several channels.

First, become associated with a local Parkinson's support group. You will learn more about your own or your family member's ailment this way than you ever thought possible, and you will have an enjoyable time.

Second, look into joining one of the national Parkinson's groups listed above. They are a major source not only of literature and information but of referrals, films, videos, lectures, groups, or whatever your needs happen to be. The newsletters published by the United Parkinson Foundation, American Parkinson Disease Association, and the Parkinson's Disease Foundation are worth the price of joining alone.

Finally, read, read, read. The following list of books and periodicals will get you started:

• Sidney Dorros, *Parkinson's: A Patient's View* (New York: Warner Books, 1981).

• Roger C. Duvoisin, *Parkinson's Disease: A Guide for Patient and Family* (New York: Raven Press, 1984).

• Richard Godwin-Austen, *The Parkinson's Disease Handbook* (Baltimore: International Health, 1984).

• J. David Grimes, Peggy A. Gray, and Kelly A. Grimes, *One Step at a Time: Problems and Answers for Patients and Health Professionals* (Ottawa: Parkinson's Society of Ottawa-Carleton, 1989).

• J. Thomas Hutton and Raye Lynne Dippel, *Caring for the Parkinson Patient: A Practical Guide* (Buffalo, New York: Prometheus Books, 1989).

• Susan B. Levin, editor, *Coping with Parkinson's Disease* (St. Louis: American Parkinson Disease Association, 1986).

• A. N. Lieberman, G. Gopinathan, A. Neophytides, and M. Goldstein, *Parkinson's Disease Handbook* (New York: The American Parkinson Disease Association, n.d.).

• "Parkinson's Disease Update Monthly." For ordering information write P.O. Box 24622, Philadelphia, PA 19111.

• Jon Robert Pierce, *Living with Parkinson's Disease or Don't Rush Me! I'm Coping As Fast As I Can* (Knoxville: Spectrum Communications, 1989).

• Gerald Stern and Andrew Lees, *Parkinson's Disease: The Facts* (Oxford, New York: Oxford University Press, 1990).

• Jan Peter Stern, *The Parkinson's Challenge: A Beginner's Guide to a Good Life in the Slow Lane.* Self-published. For ordering information write to the author, P.O. Box 1817, Santa Monica, CA 90406.

• Ivan Vaughan, *Ivan: Living with Parkinson's Disease* (New York: Farrar, Straus & Giroux, 1987).

AN OPTIMISTIC MIND

Parkinson's disease is a difficult affliction, of this there is no doubt. It is a burdening ailment, a debilitating disease. And yet, of all the serious diseases known to humankind, this one ranks high on the list of those that patients can do something about.

So if you are a parkinsonian, or if you are a caregiver for someone with the disease, do everything you can to avoid the passivity trap. Stay active. Get out of the house on a regular basis. Do your exercises, take your medications, talk to other patients, join a support group, and find out all you can. Most of all, keep a right mental attitude. As the saying goes, "An optimistic mind is a well mind."

With PD, as with any no-nonsense difficulty, the more one faces the situation squarely, actively, yet acceptingly, the better everything will seem. The more one strives to do for oneself or for the person who is being helped, the better one will feel about the world, the situation—and about oneself. Hear the final and telling words of PD patient Jan Peter Stern talking about his PD:

> Rather than reject reality and be ashamed of my tremor, I am learning to accept and even embrace challenges. I now feel more comfortable about seeing myself in the mirror, as well as about how others see me. Once I learn to retrain myself and make the conscious refinement now needed in my life, I can turn back the tide towards a more balanced, fulfilled life. This leaves my mind free to fully experience daily joys and surprises. . . . Then I can look the whole world in the eye and, when asked "How are you?" reply: "In some ways, better than ever!"[1]

NOTE

1. Jan Peter Stern, *The Parkinson's Challenge: A Beginner's Guide to a Good Life in the Slow Lane* (self-published, 1987), 26.

Appendix

A Few More Useful Resources

Free Educational Material

Free educational material is available from all major Parkinson's groups in the United States. See Chapter 15 for a listing. Especially lavish in their offerings is the American Parkinson Disease Foundation, which presently offers the following helpful books, several of which are available in languages other than English:

Basic Information About Parkinson's Disease
Parkinson's Disease Handbook
Coping with Parkinson's Disease
Home Exercises for Patients with Parkinson's Disease
Equipment and Suggestions
Speech Problems and Swallowing Problems in Parkinson's Disease
How to Start a Parkinson's Disease Community Support Group

Call the APDF to order these books at toll-free
800-223-2732.

Information on Urinary Incontinence

For information on urinary incontinence the following organization will send you copies of "Urinary Incontinence in Adults": Director of Communications, Office of Medical Applications of Research, National Institute of Health, Building 1, Room 257, Bethesda, MD 20892. Also useful is the book *Managing Incontinence* by Cheryle Gartley, published by Jamison Books, P.O. Box 738, Ottawa, IL 61350. It costs $12.95 including postage.

Consumer Information Catalog

General information on aging and medical care for the elderly is available free in the *Consumer Information Catalog*. This book provides important updates on Medicare, Medigap, health insurance, generic drugs, dietery needs of older Americans, and much more. Write to: Consumer Information Center, Pueblo, CO 81002 for a copy.

Summer Camp for PD

Every year the Parkinson Support Groups of America in Leonardtown, Maryland, in conjunction with the Sisters of Charity, run a summer camp known as Camp Maria. The camp offers a relaxing vacation geared especially for PD people, complete with swimming, canoeing, and other social recreation. For those interested, call Ida Raitano, 301-937-1545.

Information on Tranquilizers and Parkinson's Medications

Although tranquilizers certainly have a place among PD users, many patients become seriously confused trying to figure out which tranquilizers can be safely used with which PD medications. For free information, call the AARP (American Association of Retired Persons) Pharmacy Service at 703-684-0244.

Help with Dental Problems

Parkinson's patients who suffer from dry mouth often suffer from gum disease as well. For information on overall dental care, get in touch with the American Dental Association, 211 East Chicago Ave., Chicago, IL 60611.

Getting Social Security Benefits

If you are a PD person and you believe you are not getting Social Security benefits that are rightfully yours, call the National Organization of Social Security Claimants. If you qualify, they will assign you a lawyer. If you win your case, you give them 25 percent of your retroactive payments. If you lose, you pay only for their out-of-pocket expenses. Call NOSSCR, toll-free 800-431-2804, or write NOSSCR, 19 E. Central Ave., Pearl River, NY 10965.

Computer Discount Program

IBM, in conjunction with the United Cerebral Palsy Foundation and National Easter Seals, offers a computer purchase discount program for the handicapped and disabled. Those who qualify can purchase IBM Personal System/2 machines at discounts as high as 50 percent. For information, call Karen Franklin at the United Cerebral Palsy Foundation, toll-free 800-USA-5UCP, or Ann Saul at National Easter Seals, 312-243-8400.

Finding the Cheapest Medications

AARP offers "The Community Pharmacy Surveys: A How-To Kit," which is a free step-by-step kit that shows you how to comparison shop for medications in your community. The package offers sample letters to drugstores, a questionnaire, results chart, and general tips. Send your request to: Community Pharmacy Surveys (D13656), AARP Fulfillment, 1990 K Street, NW, Washington, DC 20049.

Newsletter Especially for Caregivers

The *National Well Spouse Newsletter* is written to provide caregivers with information, resources, and networking opportunities. It's catching on. For information write: National Well Spouses, Box 100, Little, Brown and Company, 205 Lexington Ave., New York, NY 10016.

Finding Out More About Home Care

If you are considering home care for yourself or for a spouse with Parkinson's, the National Association for Home Care provides free information and referrals on the subject. Call between 9 A.M. and 6 P.M. EST, Monday through Friday, at 202-547-7472.

Caregiver Self-Help

The National Self-Help Clearinghouse maintains a listing of all U.S. self-help groups and provides referrals for caregiver's specific needs. Write to: National Self-Help Clearinghouse, Graduate School University Center, City University of New York, 33 W. 42nd St., New York, NY 10036.

Index

Bu-Lax, 185
Bulk-forming laxatives, 185
Buttoners, mechanical, 198

Cadence counts, 142
Caffeine, 88, 159
Calculators, 206
Cambridge University, 111
Camp Maria, 226
Cane, 149
Car
  driving, *see* Driving
  getting out of a, 153
  insurance, 164
Carbidopa, 10, 85, 183
Carbon monoxide poisoning, 45
Caregiver
  getting help, 209–28
  newsletter for, 228
  speech of Parkinson's patient and,
    194–95
*Caring for the Parkinson Patient: A Practical
  Guide* (Hutton and Dippel), 222
Carpeting, 206
Cascara sagrada, 185
Castor oil, 185
CAT (computerized axial tomography)
  scan, 43, 49
Caudate nucleus, 108
Cenalax, 185
Chair
  getting up from a, 152–53
  sitting down, 153
Charcot, Jean-Martin, 20, 65
Chest pain, 22
Chewing gum, 178, 179
Chlorpromazine family of drugs, 45
Choking, 28, 174, 176
  Heimlich maneuver, 178, 210
  on pills, 177
Cleo, Inc., 198–207
  address, 207
Clothing
  for exercise, 133
  for sleeping, 159
  See also Dressing

Coffee, 88, 159
Cogentin, 75, 76, 78
Cogwheeling rigidity, 10, 39, 40
Colace, 185
Combs, 201
Communications
  aids to, 205–6
  See also Speech; Speech therapy;
    Telephones
"Community Pharmacy Surveys: A
  How-To Kit," 227–28
Companions, in-home, 219
Computers, discounts on, 227
Confusion as drug side effect, 91, 100,
  101
Conjunctivitis, 30
Conscious Living Foundation, 171
Constipation, 29, 77, 81, 87, 183–86
  diet, 183–84, 186
  drugs causing, 77, 81, 87, 183
  exercise, 184
  fiber, 183–84
  laxatives, 184–86
Consumer Information Catalog, 226
Consumer Information Center, 226
Cool down exercises, 124–26
Coping, 56–63
  accepting the diagnosis, 56
  knowing your resources, 60–61
  learning about Parkinson's, 58–59
  positive attitude, 62–63
  preparing for emotional ups and
    downs, 57–58
  remembering the disease is
    manageable, 56–57
  seeking counsel, 59
  understanding your medications, 61–62
  working closely with doctor, 59–60
Coping with Parkinson's Disease (Levin), 222,
  225
Corgard, 105
Cornell-UCLA scale, 51
Corpus striatum, 6, 10, 65, 84, 99, 108
Cost of medications, 68–70, 227–28
Coughing when eating, 173, 174
Counseling, 59, 60–61, 211–13
CPR, 210